The Power Of Holistic Healing Herbs: *Ancient Remedies For Modern Ailments*

Dr. Robert E. Wright

Introduction

1. Welcome and Purpose

- **Introduction to the Concept of Holistic Healing Herbs:**

In a world where the pace of life seems to quicken each day and the demands on our health become more complex, there is a growing interest in holistic healing—an approach that recognizes the interconnectedness of mind, body, and spirit. At the heart of this ancient wisdom lies the power of holistic healing herbs, offering a natural and time-tested remedy for modern ailments.

Holistic healing herbs, deeply rooted in traditional medicinal systems worldwide, have stood the test of time. Whether found in the ancient practices of Ayurveda, Traditional Chinese Medicine, Native American traditions, or other indigenous cultures, these herbs have been revered for their profound healing properties. They not only address physical symptoms but also consider the broader context of an individual's well-being.

This holistic approach acknowledges that true health extends beyond the absence of illness; it encompasses a harmonious balance between the various facets of our being. Holistic healing herbs play a pivotal role in supporting this balance, offering a diverse array of remedies for ailments that affect both the body and the mind.

As we embark on a journey to explore the power of holistic healing herbs, we delve into the rich history of their usage, blending ancient wisdom with modern scientific validation. This book aims to empower you with knowledge about essential herbs, their preparations, and their applications for common health concerns. By understanding the synergy between nature and our well-being, we open the door to a holistic lifestyle—one that embraces the healing power of herbs to promote vitality, resilience, and a profound sense of balance in our lives. Join me on this exploration of "The Power of Holistic Healing Herbs: Ancient Remedies for Modern Ailments" and discover the transformative potential that lies within the embrace of nature's healing gifts.

- **The purpose of the book: exploring ancient remedies for contemporary health issues.**

The purpose of "The Power of Holistic Healing Herbs: Ancient Remedies for Modern Ailments" is to bridge the gap between ancient wisdom and contemporary health challenges. In an era dominated by advanced medical technologies and pharmaceutical interventions, there is a growing recognition of the limitations and side effects associated with conventional approaches. This book seeks to address the evolving needs of individuals who are increasingly drawn to holistic alternatives and are curious about the healing potential embedded in traditional practices.

Key Objectives:

1. Tap into Ancient Wisdom:

- Explore the time-tested wisdom of ancient healing traditions from various cultures that have relied on the therapeutic properties of herbs for centuries.
- Showcase the accumulated knowledge that has been passed down through generations, emphasizing the efficacy of holistic approaches to health.

2. Provide Natural Solutions:

- Offer a comprehensive guide to a diverse array of herbs known for their medicinal properties.

- Present natural remedies that not only address symptoms but also target the root causes of contemporary health issues.

3. Bridge Tradition and Science:

- Validate the historical use of herbs with modern scientific research, providing readers with evidence-based insights into the effectiveness of holistic healing practices.
- Highlight the synergy between ancient wisdom and contemporary understanding, emphasizing the relevance of holistic healing in the present day.

4. Empower Readers with Knowledge:

- Empower readers to take control of their health by providing accessible information on the benefits and applications of holistic healing herbs.
- Encourage readers to make informed choices that align with their individual well-being, fostering a sense of agency and self-care.

5. Address Common Ailments:

- Specifically, target prevalent modern health issues such as stress, anxiety,

digestive problems, and immune system support.
- Offer practical solutions and insights into incorporating holistic healing practices into daily life for improved overall health and wellness.

6. Promote a Holistic Lifestyle:

- Advocate for a holistic approach to health that extends beyond symptom management to encompass mental, emotional, and spiritual well-being.
- Provide guidance on cultivating a balanced and sustainable lifestyle that integrates the power of holistic healing herbs.

By exploring ancient remedies in the context of contemporary health issues, this book aims to empower readers to embrace a holistic perspective on well-being. It invites individuals to discover the transformative potential of incorporating holistic healing herbs into their lives, promoting a harmonious and integrated approach to health in the modern world.

2. The Relevance of Holistic Healing

Holistic healing is increasingly relevant in today's world due to a shifting paradigm in how individuals approach health and well-being. The relevance of holistic healing lies in its comprehensive and interconnected approach to health, addressing not only physical symptoms but also considering mental, emotional, and spiritual aspects. Here are some key reasons why holistic healing is gaining importance:

1. Comprehensive Well-Being:

- Holistic healing recognizes that true health involves a balance between the mind, body, and spirit. It goes beyond the reductionist approach of treating isolated symptoms and focuses on promoting

overall well-being.

2. Personalized and Patient-Centered Care:

- Holistic healing emphasizes individuality, acknowledging that each person is unique. It tailors treatment plans to the specific needs and circumstances of the individual, fostering a more personalized and patient-centered approach to care.

3. Prevention and Root Cause Identification:

- Holistic healing seeks to identify and address the root causes of health issues rather than merely alleviating symptoms. By addressing the underlying imbalances, it aims to prevent the recurrence of health problems.

4. Integration of Conventional and Alternative Approaches:

- Many individuals are recognizing the value of integrating conventional medical approaches with complementary and alternative therapies. Holistic healing provides a framework for combining the strengths of both paradigms, promoting a more comprehensive and balanced approach to health care.

5. Emphasis on Lifestyle and Prevention:

- Holistic healing places a strong emphasis on lifestyle factors, including nutrition, exercise, stress management, and mindfulness. This focus on preventive measures aligns with the growing interest in maintaining health rather than simply treating illness.

6. Mind-Body Connection:

- Holistic healing acknowledges the intricate connection between the mind and body. Emotional and mental well-being are recognized as integral components of overall health, influencing physical health outcomes.

7. Patient Empowerment:

- Holistic healing empowers individuals to take an active role in their health. By providing education and encouraging self-care practices, it fosters a sense of empowerment and responsibility for one's well-being.

8. Cultural and Historical Wisdom:

- The resurgence of interest in holistic healing also stems from a recognition of the rich cultural and historical wisdom embedded in traditional healing practices. Ancient systems such as Ayurveda, Traditional Chinese Medicine, and Indigenous healing traditions offer

valuable insights into the holistic
approach to health.

9. Addressing Chronic Conditions:

- As the prevalence of chronic health conditions rises, holistic healing offers a comprehensive approach to managing and improving the quality of life for individuals dealing with long-term health challenges.

10. Growing Consumer Awareness:

- With increased access to information, consumers are becoming more aware of alternative health approaches and are seeking options beyond conventional medicine. Holistic healing aligns with this evolving awareness and desire for a more integrative approach to health.

In summary, the relevance of holistic healing lies in its holistic, patient-centered, and preventive approach, addressing the diverse and interconnected aspects of an individual's well-being in the context of today's complex health landscape.

The growing interest in holistic approaches to health.

The growing interest in holistic approaches to health reflects a broader societal shift toward a more comprehensive and integrated understanding of well-being. Several factors contribute to this increasing interest:

1. Desire for Personalization:

- Individuals are seeking personalized approaches to health that consider their unique physical, mental, and emotional needs. Holistic approaches offer customized solutions that recognize the diversity of individuals.

2. Limitations of conventional medicine:

- While conventional medicine has made significant advancements, there is a growing awareness of its limitations, particularly in addressing chronic conditions, preventing disease, and managing the side effects of certain treatments. Holistic approaches are often viewed as complementary and can fill these gaps.

3. Empowerment Through Self-Care:

- Holistic approaches empower individuals to take an active role in their health through lifestyle choices, stress management, and self-care practices. This sense of empowerment aligns with a broader cultural shift toward proactive health management.

4. Recognition of Mind-Body Connection:

- The acknowledgment of the intricate connection between mental and physical health is driving interest in holistic approaches. Many people are recognizing the impact of stress, emotions, and mental well-being on overall health.

5. Preventive Health Focus:

- Holistic approaches emphasize preventive measures, promoting overall health and well-being to avoid the development of diseases. This preventive focus resonates with individuals who are increasingly interested in maintaining good health rather than just treating illnesses.

6. Cultural and Historical Wisdom:

- Traditional healing systems, such as
  Ayurveda, Traditional Chinese Medicine,
  and Indigenous practices, offer holistic
  frameworks that have been passed down
  through generations. The growing interest
  in these systems reflects a desire to
  reconnect with cultural and historical
  wisdom.

7. Rise of Integrative Medicine:

- Integrative medicine, which combines
  conventional medical treatments with
  complementary and alternative therapies,
  is gaining acceptance. This approach
  recognizes the value of holistic practices

in conjunction with evidence-based
medicine.

8. Access to Information:

- The internet and social media have made
health information more accessible.
People are increasingly informed about
alternative therapies, herbal remedies, and
holistic practices, fueling curiosity and
interest in exploring these options.

9. Shift in Values:

- There's a broader societal shift toward
values such as sustainability, natural
living, and environmental consciousness.
Holistic approaches often align with these

values, emphasizing natural remedies,
plant-based medicine, and
environmentally friendly practices.

10. Positive Experiences and Testimonials:

- As more individuals share positive
  experiences and testimonials about the
  benefits of holistic approaches, others
  become inspired to explore these
  methods. Word-of-mouth and personal
  stories play a significant role in driving
  interest.

11. Holistic Approaches in Mainstream Culture:

- Concepts such as mindfulness,
  meditation, yoga, and herbal remedies

have become more mainstream, contributing to the normalization of holistic approaches in popular culture.

In conclusion, the growing interest in holistic approaches to health is a multifaceted phenomenon driven by a combination of individual preferences, a desire for personalized care, the limitations of conventional medicine, and a broader cultural shift toward holistic well-being. This trend is likely to continue as people seek comprehensive and integrative solutions for their health and wellness.

- **The limitations of conventional medicine and the need for complementary alternatives.**

Conventional medicine has made tremendous advancements, saving lives and alleviating suffering.

However, it also has limitations, and there is a growing recognition of the need for complementary activities to address these shortcomings. Here are some key limitations of conventional medicine:

1. Focus on Symptomatic Treatment:

- Conventional medicine often focuses on treating symptoms rather than addressing the underlying causes of health issues. This can lead to a cycle of managing symptoms without necessarily achieving long-term resolution.

2. Side Effects of Medications:

- Many pharmaceutical drugs come with potential side effects, which can range from mild discomfort to severe complications. Balancing the benefits and risks of medications is a challenge, especially for individuals with multiple health concerns.

3. Chronic Disease Management:

- Conventional medicine excels in acute care but can face challenges in managing chronic conditions. Chronic diseases often require ongoing, holistic approaches that address lifestyle factors, mental health, and preventive measures.

4. Overreliance on Pharmaceuticals:

- There is a perception of overreliance on pharmaceutical interventions, with a tendency to prescribe medications as a primary solution rather than exploring lifestyle changes or complementary therapies.

5. Limited Emphasis on Prevention:

- Conventional medicine traditionally focuses more on treating established diseases than on preventive measures. Holistic approaches, including lifestyle modifications and natural remedies, play a crucial role in preventing illnesses before they manifest.

6. Neglect of Mental and Emotional Health:

- Mental health is gaining recognition as a significant aspect of overall well-being. However, conventional medicine may sometimes overlook the intricate connection between mental and physical health, leading to incomplete treatment plans.

7. Incomplete Approach to Pain Management:

- Pain management often involves the use of painkillers, which may only provide temporary relief without addressing the root cause. Complementary activities, such as physical therapy, acupuncture, or mindfulness practices, can contribute to a more comprehensive pain management strategy.

8. Limited Individualization of Treatment:

- Conventional treatments are often standardized, and there may be a lack of personalized approaches that consider an individual's unique genetic, environmental, and lifestyle factors.

9. Cultural and Diversity Considerations:

- Conventional medicine may not always fully consider cultural and diverse perspectives on health and healing. Complementary activities, rooted in cultural practices, may offer more

inclusive and patient-centered
approaches.

10. Rise of Chronic Lifestyle-Related Illnesses:

- The prevalence of lifestyle-related illnesses, such as cardiovascular disease and type 2 diabetes, is on the rise. Conventional medicine may struggle to address the root causes, such as diet and physical activity, requiring complementary activities for comprehensive management.

Given these limitations, complementary activities become essential in providing a more holistic and patient-centered approach to health. Complementary therapies can include practices like herbal medicine, acupuncture, yoga, mindfulness, nutrition, and other lifestyle modifications. Integrating these approaches alongside conventional medicine can contribute to a more comprehensive and personalized healthcare strategy, addressing limitations and enhancing overall well-being.

Chapter 1: Understanding Holistic Healing

Holistic healing is an approach to health and wellness that considers the whole person—mind, body, spirit, and emotions—in the quest for optimal health and balance. It recognizes that these aspects of an individual are interconnected and that addressing one facet can impact the others. Here's a brief understanding of key principles within holistic healing:

1. Mind-Body Connection: Holistic healing acknowledges the profound connection between mental and physical well-being. Emotional and psychological states can influence physical health, and vice versa. Practices that promote mental and emotional balance are integral to holistic healing.

2. **Individualized and Personalized Care**: Holistic healing recognizes that each person is unique, with individual needs, preferences, and circumstances. Treatment plans are tailored to the specific characteristics and context of the individual, fostering a personalized approach to care.

3. **Preventive Focus**: Rather than solely addressing symptoms, holistic healing emphasizes preventive measures to maintain overall health. This may involve lifestyle modifications, stress management, nutritional choices, and other proactive strategies.

4. **Interconnectedness of Systems**: Holistic healing acknowledges the interconnectedness of different bodily systems. For example, digestive health can impact immune function, and emotional well-being can influence physical health. Healing approaches consider the broader context of an individual's health.

5. **Integration of Modalities**: Holistic healing often integrates a variety of therapeutic modalities, including conventional medicine, complementary therapies, and

lifestyle interventions. The goal is to create a synergistic and comprehensive approach to health.

6. **Spiritual Well-Being**: While not necessarily tied to a specific religious belief, holistic healing recognizes the importance of spiritual well-being. This may involve cultivating a sense of purpose, a connection to nature, or engaging in practices that foster spiritual growth.

7. **Natural Healing Methods**: Holistic healing often incorporates natural and alternative healing methods, such as herbal remedies, acupuncture, massage, and energy healing. These approaches aim to support the body's innate ability to heal itself.

8. **Emphasis on Holistic Lifestyle**: Beyond specific treatments, holistic healing encourages the adoption of a holistic lifestyle. This includes mindful nutrition, regular

physical activity, adequate sleep, and stress management practices to promote overall well-being.

9. **Patient Empowerment**: Holistic healing empowers individuals to take an active role in their health. Education, self-awareness, and the cultivation of healthy habits are central to this empowerment, encouraging individuals to participate in their healing journey.

10. **Recognition of Cultural Diversity**: Holistic healing is often open to diverse cultural perspectives on health and healing. It acknowledges that different cultures may have unique insights and practices that contribute to overall well-being.

In essence, holistic healing embraces a broad and interconnected view of health, seeking to address the root causes of imbalances and promote wellness at multiple levels. It encourages a proactive and integrative approach to health that goes beyond the treatment of symptoms to foster a state of holistic well-being.

1.1 Holistic Philosophy

1.1.1 The holistic approach to health

The holistic approach to health is a comprehensive and interconnected perspective that considers the entire individual—physically, mentally, emotionally, and spiritually—in the pursuit of well-being. It recognizes that these aspects of a person are interdependent and that addressing one area can have ripple effects on others. Here are key components of the holistic approach to health:

i. **Mind-Body Connection**:

- Holistic health acknowledges the intricate relationship between mental and physical well-being. Mental and emotional states can influence physical health, and vice versa. Practices such as meditation and mindfulness recognize and promote this connection.

ii. **Individualized and Person-Centered Care**:

- Holistic health recognizes that each person is unique, with individual needs, experiences, and contexts. The approach emphasizes personalized care that considers the specific circumstances, preferences, and goals of the individual.

iii. **Preventive Focus**:

- Rather than solely addressing symptoms, holistic health places a strong emphasis on preventive measures. This involves proactively adopting lifestyle choices, practices, and interventions to maintain overall health and prevent the onset of diseases.

iv. **Interconnectedness of Systems**:

- Holistic health views the body as a complex system of interconnected parts. For example, digestive health may impact immune function, and emotional well-being can affect hormonal balance. Healing is approached by considering the interplay of these systems.

v. **Integration of Modalities**:

- Holistic health integrates various therapeutic modalities, including conventional medicine, complementary and alternative therapies, and lifestyle interventions. The goal is to create a synergistic and comprehensive approach to health that addresses the root causes of imbalances.

vi. **Spiritual Well-being**:

- While not necessarily tied to religious beliefs, holistic health acknowledges the importance of spiritual well-being. This may involve cultivating a sense of purpose, connection to a higher power, or engaging in practices that foster spiritual growth.

vii. **Natural Healing Methods**:

- Holistic health often incorporates natural and alternative healing methods, such as herbal remedies, acupuncture, massage, and nutritional therapies. These approaches aim to support the body's inherent ability to heal itself and maintain balance.

viii. **Emphasis on Holistic Lifestyle**:

- Beyond specific treatments, holistic health encourages the adoption of a holistic lifestyle. This includes mindful

nutrition, regular physical activity,
sufficient rest, and stress management
practices to promote overall well-being.

ix. **Patient Empowerment**:

- Holistic health empowers individuals to actively participate in their health and healing. It involves education, self-awareness, and the cultivation of healthy habits, enabling individuals to take ownership of their well-being.

x. **Cultural Sensitivity**:

- Holistic health recognizes and respects diverse cultural perspectives on health and healing. It acknowledges that different cultures may have unique

approaches to well-being and healing

practices.

In summary, the holistic approach to health is a

philosophy that seeks to address the multifaceted nature

of well-being by considering the interconnected aspects

of an individual and promoting a balanced and integrated

approach to health care.

1.1.2 The interconnectedness of the mind, body, and spirit.

The interconnection of mind, body, and spirit is a

fundamental concept in holistic health, acknowledging

that these aspects of an individual are intricately linked

and influence one another. Here's an exploration of how

the mind, body, and spirit interconnect:

1. Mind-Body Connection:

- **Biological Basis**: Scientific research supports the bidirectional communication between the brain (mind) and the body. The nervous system, endocrine system, and immune system are interconnected, and psychological factors can impact physical health.

- **Psychosomatic Effects**: Emotional states, such as stress, anxiety, and happiness, can manifest physically. For example, chronic stress may contribute to conditions like cardiovascular disease, digestive issues, or weakened immune function.

2. Mind-Spirit Connection:

- **Consciousness and Awareness**: The mind is often considered the seat of consciousness and awareness. Spiritual practices, such as meditation or prayer, involve a heightened state of awareness that can positively impact mental well-being.

- **Mindfulness and Presence**: Spiritual practices often emphasize being present in the moment, which aligns with mindfulness principles. Mindfulness can contribute to mental clarity, emotional balance, and a sense of connection to something greater than oneself.

3. Body-Mind Connection:

- **Impact of Physical Health on Mental Well-Being**: Chronic illnesses or physical ailments can affect mental health. Pain, for example, can lead to emotional distress, anxiety, or depression. Treating physical health can positively influence mental well-being.

- **Holistic Therapies**: Body-centered therapies, such as massage, acupuncture, or yoga, recognize the intimate connection between the body and mind. These practices aim to promote physical health while simultaneously addressing mental and emotional aspects.

4. Body-Spirit Connection:

- **Physical Practices in Spirituality**: Many spiritual traditions incorporate physical practices, such as rituals, dance, or yoga. These activities are seen as a means of connecting with the divine or transcendent and may have positive effects on both the body and spiritual well-being.

- **Wellness and Spiritual Alignment**: Maintaining physical health is often considered a form of honoring the spiritual self. Practices like mindful eating, exercise, and rest contribute to overall well-being and can be viewed as spiritual acts.

5. Spirit-Mind Connection:

- **Inner Wisdom and Intuition**: The spirit is often associated with a deeper sense of inner wisdom or intuition. Spiritual practices can enhance one's ability to access this wisdom, contributing to mental clarity and decision-making.

- **Guidance in Times of Challenge**: Spiritual beliefs and practices can provide a source of strength and guidance during challenging times, offering a framework for coping with stress, grief, or existential questions.

In summary, the mind, body, and spirit form an integrated system where changes or influences in one aspect can have profound effects on the others. Holistic health approaches aim to promote balance and harmony among these interconnected elements, recognizing the importance of addressing the whole person for optimal well-being. Practices that nourish the mind, nurture the body, and connect with the spirit contribute to a holistic and integrated approach to health.

1.2 History of Holistic Healing

1.2.1 Historical roots of holistic healing

The historical roots of holistic healing can be traced back to ancient civilizations and diverse cultural traditions that recognized the interconnectedness of various aspects of human existence. Here is a brief overview of the historical roots of holistic healing:

1. Ayurveda (Ancient India):

- ***Time Period***: Ayurveda, the traditional system of medicine in India, has roots dating back over 5,000 years.

- ***Philosophy***: Ayurveda emphasizes balance in bodily systems, incorporating elements such as diet, herbal medicine, yoga, and meditation to promote holistic health.

- ***Interconnectedness***: It recognizes the interdependence of mind, body, and spirit and considers the individual's unique constitution (dosha) in health and disease.

2. Traditional Chinese Medicine (TCM):
- ***Time Period***: TCM has evolved over several millennia, with its roots traced back to the Shang Dynasty (16th to 11th century BCE).

- ***Philosophy***: TCM views the body as a system of interconnected energy pathways (meridians). Acupuncture, herbal medicine, Qi Gong, and Tai Chi are integral components aiming to balance the flow of energy (Qi) for overall well-being.

3. Greek Medicine (Hippocratic Tradition):

- ***Time Period***: The Hippocratic tradition, named after the ancient Greek physician Hippocrates (460–370 BCE), emphasized a holistic approach to health.

- ***Philosophy***: It viewed the body as a complex system influenced by environmental factors and advocated for a balance of the four humors (blood, phlegm, black bile, and yellow bile) for good health.

4. Indigenous Healing Traditions:

- ***Time Period***: Indigenous healing practices vary widely across cultures and have ancient roots that predate recorded history.

- ***Philosophy***: Indigenous healing often incorporates a deep connection to nature, rituals, and herbal remedies. Practices are passed down through oral traditions and involve a holistic understanding of the individual's relationship to the community and the environment.

5. Islamic Medicine:

- ***Time Period***: Islamic medicine flourished from the 7th to the 13th centuries.

- ***Philosophy***: Islamic scholars integrated Greek, Roman, and Indian medical knowledge, emphasizing a holistic approach to health. The

Persian polymath Avicenna's "Canon of Medicine" is a notable work from this tradition.

6. Herbalism in Europe:

- *Time Period*: Herbalism has roots in ancient European cultures, and its practices persisted through the Middle Ages and Renaissance.

- *Philosophy*: European herbalism relied on the use of plants for medicinal purposes, considering the holistic impact of herbs on the body. Wise women and healers were often central to these traditions.

7. Holism in the 19th and 20th Centuries:

- *Time Period*: The concept of holism gained renewed attention in the 19th and 20th centuries.

- *Philosophy*: Holistic healing principles were revisited, with a focus on integrating mind, body, and spirit. Holistic pioneers, such as Dr. Andrew Weil and Dr. Rachel Carson, contributed to the revival of holistic approaches in modern times.

These historical roots collectively laid the foundation for contemporary holistic healing practices. While the specific philosophies and methods may vary, the underlying principle of addressing the whole person for health and well-being remains a common thread in holistic traditions around the world.

1.2.2 Ancient civilizations and their use of herbs for medicinal purposes

Various ancient civilizations recognized the therapeutic properties of herbs and integrated them into their medical practices for healing and well-being. Here is an exploration of how some ancient civilizations used herbs for medicinal purposes:

1. Ancient Egypt:

- *Time Period*: 3000 BCE to 30 BCE

- *Herbal Practices*: Ancient Egyptians used a wide array of herbs for medicinal purposes. They recorded their knowledge on medical papyri, such as the Ebers Papyrus, which detailed herbal remedies for various ailments. Herbs like aloe vera, garlic, and myrrh were commonly employed.

2. Ancient China:

- *Time Period*: 2700 BCE onwards

- **Herbal Practices**: Traditional Chinese Medicine (TCM) has a rich history of using herbs for therapeutic purposes. The "Shennong Ben Cao Jing," one of the earliest Chinese herbals, documented hundreds of herbs and their properties. Ginseng, ginger, and licorice are examples of herbs extensively used in TCM.

3. Ancient India (Ayurveda):

- *Time Period*: Over 5,000 years

- *Herbal Practices*: Ayurveda, the traditional system of medicine in India, emphasizes the use of herbs for promoting balance and preventing disease. Herbs such as turmeric, neem, and ashwagandha play a significant role in Ayurvedic formulations.

4. Ancient Greece:

- *Time Period*: 5th century BCE onwards

- *Herbal Practices*: Hippocrates, often regarded as the "Father of Medicine," emphasized the use of herbs in his teachings. The Greeks used herbs like chamomile, thyme, and oregano for their medicinal properties. The concept of the four humors influenced herbal prescriptions.

5. Ancient Rome:

- *Time Period*: 509 BCE to 476 CE

- *Herbal Practices*: Roman medicine inherited much from Greek traditions. The physician Galen, influenced by Hippocrates, made significant contributions to herbal medicine. Herbs such as sage, rosemary, and mint were commonly used for various health purposes.

6. Ancient Mesopotamia:

- *Time Period*: 3500 BCE to 539 BCE

- *Herbal Practices*: The ancient Mesopotamians, including the Babylonians and Assyrians, utilized herbs for medicinal purposes. Clay tablets with medical inscriptions detail the use of herbs like

myrrh, opium poppy, and saffron for healing.

7. Indigenous Cultures (e.g., Native Americans):
- **Time Period**: Varied, with continuous practices

  to the present

- *Herbal Practices*: Indigenous cultures

  worldwide, including Native American tribes,

  have a rich tradition of herbal medicine. Plants

  like echinacea, yarrow, and sage were used for

  their medicinal properties. Knowledge was often

  passed down through oral traditions.

8. Islamic Golden Age:
- *Time Period*: 8th to 14th centuries

- *Herbal Practices*: During the Islamic Golden

  Age, scholars like Avicenna (Ibn Sina)

  contributed significantly to herbal medicine.

Avicenna's "Canon of Medicine" included extensive information on herbs and their medicinal properties.

9. Ancient Japan:

- *Time Period*: From ancient times

- *Herbal Practices*: Traditional Japanese medicine, influenced by Chinese medicine, incorporated the use of herbs. Kampo medicine, a Japanese adaptation of Chinese herbal medicine, includes herbs like ginger, licorice, and cinnamon.

These ancient civilizations recognized the therapeutic potential of herbs and integrated them into holistic approaches to health. The accumulated knowledge from these traditions has influenced contemporary herbal medicine and holistic healing practices.

Chapter 2: The Power of Herbs

The power of herbs lies in their natural compounds and properties, which have been utilized for centuries for various health and wellness purposes. Here are some aspects of the power of herbs:

1. Medicinal Properties:

- **Anti-Inflammatory**: Many herbs possess anti-inflammatory properties, helping to reduce inflammation in the body. Examples include turmeric, ginger, and boswellia.
- **Antioxidant**: Herbs like rosemary, oregano, and green tea are rich in antioxidants, which can neutralize free radicals and support overall health.
- **Adaptogenic**: Adaptogenic herbs like ashwagandha and rhodiola help the body adapt to stress and maintain balance.

2. Traditional Healing Wisdom:

- **Ancient Remedies**: Herbs have been a fundamental part of traditional medicine systems worldwide, such as Ayurveda, Traditional Chinese Medicine (TCM), and Indigenous healing practices.

3. Holistic Approach:

- **Mind-Body Connection**: Many herbs address not only physical symptoms but also contribute to mental and emotional well-being, emphasizing a holistic approach to health.

4. Nutrient Density:

- **Vitamins and Minerals**: Herbs are often rich in vitamins and minerals, contributing to nutritional support. For example, parsley is high in vitamin K, while cilantro provides antioxidants.

5. Supportive of Various Health Conditions:

- **Immune Support**: Herbs like echinacea, garlic, and astragalus are known for their immune-boosting properties.
- **Digestive Health**: Peppermint, ginger, and fennel are herbs that can support digestive health and ease discomfort.

6. Versatility:

- **Culinary Uses**: Many herbs are used in cooking to enhance the flavor of dishes. Culinary herbs like basil, thyme, and rosemary can also offer health benefits.

7. Preventive Health:

- **Preventive Properties**: Regular consumption of certain herbs is believed to contribute to preventive health measures, supporting the body in avoiding imbalances and diseases.

8. Holistic Practices:

- **Herbalism**: Herbalism is the practice of using plants for medicinal purposes. Herbalists often consider the whole person and aim to address the root cause of health issues.

9. Research Support:

- **Scientific Studies**: Research studies increasingly explore the therapeutic potential of herbs, providing evidence for their efficacy in various health conditions.

10. Personalized Healing:

- **Individualized Approaches**: Herbs allow for personalized and individualized approaches to health, recognizing that different individuals may respond differently to herbal interventions.

11. Cultural Significance:

- **Cultural and Spiritual Significance**: Many herbs hold cultural and spiritual significance, contributing to a sense of connection and well-being in various communities.

12. Accessible and Sustainable:

- **Accessibility**: Herbs are often readily available, making them accessible to a wide range of people.
- **Sustainability**: Growing and using herbs can be part of sustainable and environmentally friendly practices.

13. Complementary to Conventional Medicine:

- **Complementary Healing**: Herbs can complement conventional medical treatments, providing additional support and addressing aspects beyond the scope of pharmaceutical interventions.

While herbs can be powerful allies in supporting health, it's important to approach their use with respect and, when needed, seek guidance from qualified healthcare professionals or herbalists. The power of herbs is best harnessed when integrated into a holistic and well-balanced lifestyle.

2.1 Herbs in Traditional Medicine

2.1.1 Different traditional healing systems

Various traditional healing systems have evolved over

centuries, offering unique approaches to health and well-being. Here's an exploration of some prominent

traditional healing systems:

1. Ayurveda:

- ***Origin***: Ancient India (over 5,000 years old)

- ***Philosophy***: Ayurveda emphasizes balance in bodily systems and the interconnectedness of mind, body, and spirit. It classifies individuals into three doshas (Vata, Pitta, Kapha) and prescribes personalized approaches to diet, lifestyle, and herbal remedies.

- ***Methods***: Herbal medicine, diet and nutrition, yoga, meditation, massage (Abhyanga), and detoxification (Panchakarma).

2. Traditional Chinese Medicine (TCM):

- ***Origin***: Ancient China (over 2,500 years old)

- *Philosophy*: TCM views the body as a system of interconnected energy pathways (meridians) through which Qi (life force) flows. The balance of Yin and Yang is central to health. TCM uses acupuncture, herbal medicine, cupping, Qi Gong, and dietary therapy.

- *Methods*: Acupuncture, herbal medicine, cupping therapy, moxibustion, Qi Gong, and Tui Na (therapeutic massage).

3. Unani Medicine:

- *Origin*: Ancient Greece, Persia, and India; developed during the Islamic Golden Age

- *Philosophy*: Unani medicine is based on the principles of balancing the four humors (blood, phlegm, black bile, yellow bile). It incorporates elements of Greek, Arabic, and Persian medicine, emphasizing the body's natural healing processes.

- *Methods*: Herbal medicine, dietary recommendations, cupping therapy, and lifestyle modifications.

4. Traditional African Medicine:

- *Origin*: Diverse practices across the African continent

- *Philosophy*: Traditional African medicine varies widely among different ethnic groups. Practices often involve the use of medicinal plants, rituals, and the guidance of traditional healers. Spiritual and community aspects are integral to healing.

- *Methods*: Herbal remedies, divination, rituals, and the expertise of traditional healers.

5. Native American Medicine:

- *Origin*: Indigenous cultures of North and South America

- *Philosophy*: Native American medicine emphasizes the interconnectedness of nature and humans. Healing practices involve herbal medicine, rituals, ceremonies, and a holistic approach to well-being.

- *Methods*: Herbal remedies, sweat lodges, smudging, and rituals guided by traditional healers.

6. Siddha Medicine:

- *Origin*: Ancient Tamil civilization (Southern India)

- *Philosophy*: Siddha medicine is rooted in the concept of balancing the three doshas (Vata, Pitta, and Kapha) and achieving harmony in the body. It incorporates herbal medicine, dietary

practices, yoga, and meditation.

- *Methods*: Herbal remedies, dietary guidelines,
  yoga, meditation, and detoxification practices.

7. Kampo Medicine:

- *Origin*: Japan (influenced by Traditional Chinese
  Medicine)

- *Philosophy*: Kampo medicine adapted Chinese
  medicine principles to Japanese culture. It
  focuses on restoring the balance of Qi and
  incorporates herbal remedies, acupuncture, and
  dietary recommendations.

- *Methods*: Herbal medicine, acupuncture, and
  dietary therapy.

8. Hopi Medicine:

- ***Origin***: Hopi Native American tribe
  (Southwestern United States)

- ***Philosophy***: Hopi medicine integrates
  spirituality, rituals, and herbal knowledge.
  Healing practices involve the use of ceremonial
  herbs, rituals guided by spiritual leaders, and a
  connection to the spiritual world.

- ***Methods***: Herbal remedies, rituals, and
  ceremonies led by spiritual leaders.

These traditional healing systems showcase the diversity
of approaches to health and well-being, highlighting the
importance of personalized, holistic care that considers
the interconnected aspects of an individual's life. Each
system reflects a deep understanding of the relationships
between the body, mind, spirit, and the natural
environment.

2.1.2 The central role of herbs in these systems.

Herbs play a central and foundational role in various traditional healing systems, serving as key components for promoting health, preventing illness, and supporting overall well-being. Here's an exploration of the central role of herbs in several traditional healing systems:

1. Ayurveda:
- ***Role of Herbs***: Ayurveda relies extensively on herbal medicine. Herbs are categorized based on their tastes, qualities, and effects on the doshas. They are used to balance doshas, strengthen tissues, promote digestion, and address specific health concerns.

- ***Examples***: Turmeric for its anti-inflammatory properties, Ashwagandha for stress adaptation, and Triphala for digestive support.

2. Traditional Chinese Medicine (TCM):

- ***Role of Herbs***: Herbal medicine is one of the key modalities in TCM. Formulas often consist of multiple herbs working synergistically to balance Qi, Yin, and Yang. Herbs are categorized by taste, temperature, and specific actions.

- ***Examples***: Ginseng for energy and vitality, Astragalus for immune support, and Ginkgo Biloba for cognitive function.

3. Unani Medicine:

- ***Role of Herbs***: Unani medicine places a strong emphasis on herbal remedies. Herbs are selected to balance the four humors, strengthen organs,

and address specific imbalances. Formulations
often include a combination of herbs.

- *Examples*: Black seed (Nigella sativa) for
  respiratory health, Amla (Indian gooseberry) for
  digestion, and Safed musli for vitality.

4. Traditional African Medicine:

- *Role of Herbs*: Traditional African medicine
  relies heavily on the use of medicinal plants.
  Herbs are selected based on local knowledge, and
  the guidance of traditional healers often involves
  the spiritual and cultural context of the
  community.

- *Examples*: Rooibos for digestive health, African
  potato for immune support, and Sutherlandia
  frutescens for various ailments.

5. Native American Medicine:

- ***Role of Herbs***: Herbal remedies are integral to Native American healing practices. Plants are seen as allies with spiritual significance, used for physical and spiritual healing. Rituals often involve the use of specific herbs.

- ***Examples***: Sage for purification, Sweetgrass for ceremonial purposes, and Yarrow for various medicinal properties.

6. Siddha Medicine:

- ***Role of Herbs***: Siddha medicine places a significant emphasis on herbal remedies to balance doshas and promote overall health. Herbal formulations are designed to address specific imbalances and support the body's natural healing processes.

- *Examples*: Triphala for digestive health, Brahmi for cognitive function, and Guggul for joint support.

7. Kampo Medicine:

- ***Role of Herbs***: Kampo medicine relies on herbal formulas derived from Traditional Chinese Medicine principles. Herbs are selected to address specific patterns of disharmony in the body and restore balance.

- *Examples*: Keishibukuryogan for menstrual disorders, Hochuekkito for immune support, and Ninjinyoeito for fatigue.

8. Hopi Medicine:

- ***Role of Herbs***: Herbs are an essential component of Hopi medicine, often used in ceremonial and ritual contexts. They are believed to have spiritual significance and are employed for physical and spiritual healing.

- ***Examples***: Sage for purification, Cedar for ceremonial use, and Tobacco in rituals.

In these traditional healing systems, herbs are not only valued for their biochemical properties but also for their energetic qualities, spiritual significance, and cultural context. They are integrated into comprehensive healing practices that consider the whole person and the interconnected aspects of health.

2.2 Modern Scientific Validation

2.2.1 Scientific studies supporting the efficacy of herbal remedies

Scientific studies investigating the efficacy of herbal remedies have grown in recent years, providing valuable insights into the potential health benefits of various medicinal plants. It's important to note that while many studies show promising results, not all herbal remedies have undergone extensive research, and more studies are needed to establish their effectiveness. Here are some examples of scientific studies supporting the efficacy of certain herbal remedies:

1. Turmeric (Curcuma longa):
- **Active Compound**: Curcumin
- **Scientific Evidence**:
  - Numerous studies have investigated the anti-inflammatory and antioxidant properties of curcumin in turmeric.
  - Research suggests potential benefits in managing conditions like osteoarthritis,

rheumatoid arthritis, and inflammatory

bowel diseases.

2. Ginger (Zingiber officinale):
- **Active Compounds**: Gingerol, shogaol

- **Scientific Evidence**:

  - Studies have shown the anti-nausea

    properties of ginger, making it effective

    for nausea associated with pregnancy,

    chemotherapy, and surgery.

  - Ginger has demonstrated anti-

    inflammatory effects, potentially

    beneficial for conditions like

    osteoarthritis.

3. Echinacea (Echinacea spp.):
- **Active Compounds**: Alkamides, polysaccharides

- **Scientific Evidence**:

- Some studies suggest that echinacea may
  help reduce the severity and duration of
  colds.

- Research indicates potential
  immunomodulatory effects, supporting
  the immune system.

4. Ginkgo Biloba:
- **Active Compounds**: Flavonoids, terpenoids

- **Scientific Evidence**:

  - Studies have explored ginkgo biloba's
    potential in improving cognitive function
    and memory, especially in age-related
    cognitive decline.

  - Ginkgo biloba has been investigated for
    its antioxidant and anti-inflammatory
    properties.

5. St. John's Wort (Hypericum perforatum):
- **Active Compounds**: Hypericin, hyperforin

- **Scientific Evidence**:

  - Research has suggested that St. John's Wort may be effective in treating mild to moderate depression.

  - The herb has been studied for its potential as an antidepressant, with effects on neurotransmitters.

6. Garlic (Allium sativum):
- **Active Compounds**: Allicin, alliin

- **Scientific Evidence**:

  - Garlic has demonstrated cardiovascular benefits, including the potential to lower blood pressure and reduce cholesterol levels.

- Studies have explored its anti-inflammatory and antimicrobial properties.

7. Saw Palmetto (Serenoa repens):
- **Active Compounds**: Fatty acids, sterols

- **Scientific Evidence**:

    - Saw palmetto has been studied for its potential in managing symptoms of benign prostatic hyperplasia (BPH) by inhibiting the activity of certain hormones.

    - Research has explored its anti-inflammatory effects on the prostate.

8. Milk Thistle (Silybum marianum):
- **Active Compounds**: Silymarin

- **Scientific Evidence**:

- Studies have investigated the hepatoprotective effects of milk thistle, particularly in liver diseases.

- Silymarin has been studied for its antioxidant and anti-inflammatory properties.

9. Aloe Vera:

- **Active Compounds**: Polysaccharides, anthraquinones

- **Scientific Evidence**:

  - Aloe vera has been studied for its potential in wound healing and skin conditions, attributed to its anti-inflammatory and antimicrobial properties.

- Research suggests potential benefits for
  conditions like psoriasis and dermatitis.

10. Peppermint (Mentha × piperita):

- **Active Compounds**: Menthol, menthone

- **Scientific Evidence**:

  - Peppermint oil has been studied for its efficacy in relieving symptoms of irritable bowel syndrome (IBS), including abdominal pain and discomfort.

  - Research suggests potential antimicrobial and analgesic effects.

While these studies provide evidence supporting the efficacy of certain herbal remedies, it's crucial to approach herbal medicine with caution. Individual responses to herbs can vary, and interactions with medications or existing health conditions should be considered. Always consult with a healthcare professional before incorporating herbal remedies into your health regimen, especially if you are pregnant, nursing, or taking medications. Additionally, ongoing research is essential to further validate the efficacy and safety of herbal remedies.

2.2.2 Common misconceptions about holistic medicine

Holistic medicine, with its emphasis on treating the whole person and addressing multiple aspects of well-being, is often subject to various misconceptions. Addressing these misconceptions is important for a clearer understanding of holistic approaches to health. Here are some common misconceptions about holistic medicine:

1. Holistic Medicine is "Alternative" or "Unproven":

- **Misconception**: Some people believe that holistic medicine is synonymous with alternative or unproven therapies.

- **Clarification**: Holistic medicine encompasses a broad range of approaches, including both traditional and evidence-based practices. Many holistic modalities have been studied and

integrated into conventional healthcare.

Examples include mindfulness-based stress

reduction, acupuncture, and certain herbal

remedies.

2. Holistic Medicine Rejects Conventional Medicine:

- **Misconception**: There's a perception that holistic

  medicine is opposed to or rejects conventional

  medical treatments.

- **Clarification**: Holistic medicine often

  complements conventional medicine. It

  emphasizes an integrative approach that

  considers the benefits of both conventional

  treatments and holistic practices. Collaboration

  between healthcare providers from different

modalities is increasingly recognized for comprehensive patient care.

3. All "Natural" or "Herbal" Means Safe:

- **Misconception**: Assuming that because a remedy is natural or herbal, it is safe and without side effects.

- **Clarification**: Natural does not always mean harmless. Herbs can have potent effects and may interact with medications or exacerbate certain health conditions. It's crucial to consult with a healthcare professional before using herbal remedies, especially in conjunction with other treatments.

4. Holistic Medicine Is Only About "Mind-Body" Approaches:

- **Misconception**: Holistic medicine is often equated solely with mind-body practices like meditation, yoga, or mindfulness.

- **Clarification**: While mind-body practices are integral, holistic medicine encompasses a broader spectrum. It includes nutrition, herbal medicine, physical therapies, spiritual practices, and lifestyle modifications. The emphasis is on addressing physical, mental, emotional, and spiritual aspects.

5. Holistic Approaches Are Slow or Ineffective:

- **Misconception**: Some may believe that holistic approaches take longer to show results or are less effective than conventional treatments.

- **Clarification**: The effectiveness of holistic approaches varies depending on the individual,

the condition, and the specific modality. Some
holistic practices can provide rapid relief, while
others may require time for sustained benefits.
Holistic approaches are often focused on
preventive measures and long-term well-being.

6. Holistic Medicine Ignores Scientific Evidence:

- **Misconception**: A common misconception is
  that holistic practitioners dismiss scientific
  evidence.

- **Clarification**: Many holistic practices are
  evidence-based, and the field encourages
  rigorous scientific inquiry. However, some
  traditional practices may lack extensive scientific
  validation. Holistic medicine promotes an open-
  minded and individualized approach, combining

evidence-based practices with an understanding
of the limitations of some traditional knowledge.

7. Holistic Medicine Is Only for Chronic Conditions:

- **Misconception**: Holistic approaches are often thought to be applicable only for chronic or long-term conditions.

- **Clarification**: Holistic medicine is relevant for both prevention and management of chronic conditions as well as acute issues. It promotes overall well-being, and individuals can benefit from holistic practices regardless of their health status.

8. Holistic Medicine Is Exclusively "New Age" or Spiritual:

- **Misconception**: Holistic medicine is sometimes associated exclusively with New Age spirituality.

- **Clarification**: While spiritual aspects may be included, holistic medicine is not limited to any specific religious or spiritual belief. It accommodates diverse cultural and individual perspectives and focuses on providing care that aligns with each person's values and preferences.

9. Holistic Medicine Is Expensive:

- **Misconception**: There's a perception that holistic medicine is more costly than conventional care.

- **Clarification**: The cost of holistic medicine can vary, and many practices, such as lifestyle modifications, nutrition, and self-care, can be cost-effective. Some complementary therapies may be covered by insurance, and community resources may offer affordable holistic services.

10. Holistic Medicine Is a "Cure-All":

- **Misconception**: Holistic medicine is sometimes seen as a universal cure for all ailments.
- **Clarification**: Holistic approaches acknowledge individual differences and emphasize personalized care. While they can contribute to overall well-being, they may not be a cure for every condition. Holistic medicine encourages a comprehensive, integrative approach rather than a one-size-fits-all solution.

Understanding these misconceptions helps foster a more accurate and nuanced view of holistic medicine. Like any approach to health, it requires thoughtful consideration, collaboration with healthcare professionals, and an individualized approach based on the unique needs and circumstances of each person.

Chapter 3: Building Your Holistic Toolkit

Building a holistic toolkit involves integrating practices, habits, and resources that support overall well-being—addressing the mind, body, and spirit. Here are key elements to consider when building your holistic toolkit:

1. Mindful Practices:

- **Meditation**: Cultivate a regular meditation practice to quiet the mind, reduce stress, and enhance mental clarity.
- **Mindful Breathing**: Practice deep breathing exercises to promote relaxation and focus.

2. Herbal Remedies:

- **Teas and Infusions**: Explore herbal teas for various health benefits. Chamomile for relaxation, peppermint for digestion, and ginger for immune support are excellent choices.
- **Tinctures and Extracts**: Consider herbal tinctures for concentrated and convenient herbal remedies.

3. Nutrient-Rich Diet:

- **Whole Foods**: Prioritize a diet rich in whole foods, emphasizing fruits, vegetables, lean proteins, and whole grains.
- **Herb-Infused Cooking**: Incorporate fresh herbs into your meals for added flavor and health benefits.

4. Physical Activity:

- **Exercise Routine**: Establish a regular exercise routine that includes both cardiovascular and strength-training exercises.
- **Mindful Movement**: Explore mindful practices like yoga or tai chi for both physical and mental well-being.

5. Sleep Hygiene:

- **Sleep Rituals**: Create a calming bedtime routine, including activities like reading, gentle stretching, or practicing gratitude.
- **Herbal Sleep Aids**: Consider herbs like valerian or chamomile for their calming effects.

6. Holistic Therapies:

- **Acupuncture**: Explore acupuncture for its potential benefits in balancing energy and promoting overall health.
- **Massage Therapy**: Regular massages can aid in relaxation and reduce muscle tension.

7. Emotional Wellness:

- **Journaling**: Reflect on your thoughts and feelings through journaling to enhance emotional awareness.
- **Therapeutic Practices**: Engage in therapy or counseling to address emotional and psychological well-being.

8. Nature Connection:

- **Forest Bathing**: Spend time in nature, practicing shinrin-yoku or forest bathing, to reduce stress and promote well-being.
- **Gardening**: Cultivate a garden or indoor plants for a sense of connection with nature.

9. Social Connections:

- **Quality Relationships**: Nurture meaningful connections with friends and family for emotional support.
- **Community Involvement**: Engage in community activities to foster a sense of belonging.

10. Holistic Education:

- **Reading and Learning**: Continuously educate yourself on holistic health practices, herbalism, and mindfulness.

- **Workshops and Courses**: Attend workshops or courses on holistic well-being to deepen your understanding.

11. Spiritual Practices:

- **Mindful Prayer or Meditation**: Integrate spiritual practices that resonate with your beliefs.
- **Connection with Higher Purpose**: Cultivate a sense of purpose and connection to something greater than yourself.

12. Stress Management:

- **Stress-Reducing Activities**: Identify stressors and incorporate activities such as art, music, or hobbies for relaxation.
- **Herbs for Stress Relief**: Explore adaptogenic herbs like ashwagandha or holy basil.

13. Holistic Healthcare:

- **Integrative Medicine**: Consider consulting with integrative healthcare professionals who understand both conventional and holistic approaches.
- **Regular Check-Ups**: Maintain regular check-ups with healthcare providers for a comprehensive view of your health.

14. Digital Detox:

- **Screen-Free Time**: Schedule periods without digital devices to reduce information overload and promote mental clarity.

- **Mindful Technology Use**: Practice mindful use of technology, avoiding excessive screen time.

Building your holistic toolkit is a personal and evolving process. Regularly assess your needs, preferences, and experiences to refine and expand your toolkit for optimal well-being. Remember, the key is to approach holistic living with openness, curiosity, and a commitment to self-care.

3.1 Essential Herbs for Holistic Healing

3.1.1 A selection of powerful herbs

Here's an introduction to a selection of powerful herbs, each known for its unique properties and potential health benefits:

1. Turmeric (Curcuma longa):
- **Active Compound**: Curcumin
- **Benefits**:

- Powerful anti-inflammatory and antioxidant properties.
- Potential support for joint health.
- Studies suggest benefits for digestive health.

2. Ginger (Zingiber officinale):

- **Active Compounds**: Gingerol, shogaol
- **Benefits**:
    - Anti-nausea properties, especially helpful for motion sickness.
    - Anti-inflammatory effects, potentially beneficial for joint health.
    - May aid digestion and alleviate gastrointestinal discomfort.

3. Garlic (Allium sativum):

- **Active Compounds**: Allicin, alliin
- **Benefits**:
    - Cardiovascular support, including potential blood pressure regulation.
    - Antimicrobial properties, aiding in immune health.
    - Antioxidant effects, supporting overall well-being.

4. Ashwagandha (Withania somnifera):

- **Active Compounds**: Withanolides
- **Benefits**:
    - Adaptogenic herb for stress adaptation and resilience.

- Potential to support adrenal health.
- Studies suggest benefits for cognitive function.

5. Echinacea (Echinacea spp.):

- **Active Compounds**: Alkamides, polysaccharides
- **Benefits**:
    - Immune system support, potentially reducing the severity and duration of colds.
    - Antioxidant properties contributing to overall health.

6. Ginkgo Biloba:

- **Active Compounds**: Flavonoids, terpenoids
- **Benefits**:
    - Cognitive support, potentially improving memory and concentration.
    - Circulatory support, promoting healthy blood flow.
    - Antioxidant effects for overall well-being.

7. Holy Basil (Ocimum sanctum):

- **Active Compounds**: Eugenol, rosmarinic acid
- **Benefits**:
    - Adaptogenic herb for stress management.
    - Potential immune system support.
    - Antioxidant properties for overall health.

8. Milk Thistle (Silybum marianum):

- **Active Compounds**: Silymarin

- **Benefits**:
  - Hepatoprotective effects, supporting liver health.
  - Antioxidant properties for overall well-being.
  - Potential benefits for digestive health.

9. Peppermint (Mentha × piperita):

- **Active Compounds**: Menthol, menthone
- **Benefits**:
  - Digestive support, alleviating symptoms like indigestion and bloating.
  - Potential for headache relief and respiratory health.
  - Antimicrobial properties for oral health.

10. Rhodiola Rosea:

- **Active Compounds**: Rosavins, salidrosides
- **Benefits**:

- Adaptogenic herb for stress management and mental fatigue.

- Potential support for mood and emotional well-being.

- Studies suggest benefits for physical endurance.

These herbs have a long history of traditional use and are increasingly studied for their potential health benefits. While incorporating herbs into your health regimen, it's essential to consult with a healthcare professional, especially if you have existing health conditions or are taking medications, to ensure safety and efficacy. Additionally, individual responses to herbs can vary, and it's important to pay attention to how your body responds to any new supplement or remedy.

3.1.2 Medicinal properties and additional applications of the mentioned powerful herbs:

1. Turmeric (Curcuma longa):

- **Medicinal Properties**:
  - *Anti-inflammatory and antioxidant*:
    - Effective in reducing inflammation, making it beneficial for conditions like arthritis and inflammatory bowel diseases.
    - Potent antioxidant properties help combat oxidative stress in the body.
  - *Anticancer Potential*:
    - Studies suggest curcumin, the active compound in turmeric, may have anti-cancer properties by inhibiting the growth of cancer cells.
  - *Brain Health*:
    - Emerging research indicates potential benefits for neurodegenerative conditions, with curcumin crossing the blood-brain barrier.

- *Heart Health*:
  - May improve endothelial function and reduce the risk factors associated with heart disease.

2. Ginger (Zingiber officinale):

- **Medicinal Properties**:
  - *Anti-nausea and Anti-inflammatory*:
    - Known for relieving nausea and vomiting, including those associated with pregnancy, chemotherapy, and surgery.
    - Demonstrates anti-inflammatory effects, potentially aiding in conditions like osteoarthritis.
  - *Digestive Health*:
    - Facilitates digestion and helps alleviate indigestion and bloating.
  - *Pain Relief*:
    - May have analgesic properties, providing relief from various types of pain.
  - *Antimicrobial Effects*:
    - Exhibits antimicrobial properties that may help combat infections.

3. Garlic (Allium sativum):

- **Medicinal Properties**:
  - *Cardiovascular Support*:
    - Studies suggest garlic can lower blood pressure and cholesterol

levels, reducing the risk of
cardiovascular diseases.
- *Immune System Modulation*:
  - Known for its immune-boosting
    properties, helping the body fight
    off infections.
- *Anti-cancer Potential*:
  - Some research indicates potential
    anti-cancer effects, especially in
    preventing certain types of cancer.
- *Detoxification*:
  - Supports the body's natural
    detoxification processes,
    particularly in the liver.

4. Ashwagandha (Withania somnifera):

- **Medicinal Properties**:
  - *Adaptogenic and Anti-stress*:
    - Helps the body adapt to stress and
      promotes overall resilience.
  - *Cognitive Function*:
    - Emerging research suggests
      benefits for cognitive function,
      memory, and neuroprotection.
  - *Endocrine Support*:
    - Supports hormonal balance,
      particularly in conditions related
      to stress.
  - *Anti-anxiety and antidepressants*:
    - May have anxiolytic and
      antidepressant effects.

5. Echinacea (Echinacea spp.):

- **Medicinal Properties**:
    - *Immune System Support*:
        - Enhances the activity of the immune system, potentially reducing the severity and duration of colds.
    - *Anti-inflammatory*:
        - Contains compounds with anti-inflammatory effects.
    - *Antiviral Properties*:
        - May have antiviral effects against certain respiratory viruses.
    - *Wound Healing*:
        - Traditionally used for its wound-healing properties.

6. Ginkgo Biloba:

- **Medicinal Properties**:
    - *Cognitive Enhancement*:
        - Improves memory, concentration, and cognitive function, especially in age-related cognitive decline.
    - *Peripheral Circulation*:
        - Enhances blood flow to peripheral tissues, potentially benefiting conditions like intermittent claudication.
    - *Antioxidant Effects*:
        - Exhibits antioxidant properties, protecting cells from oxidative damage.

- *Vision Health*:
  - Some evidence suggests a role in supporting vision and eye health.

7. Holy Basil (Ocimum sanctum):

- **Medicinal Properties**:
  - *Adaptogenic and Anti-stress*:
    - Helps the body adapt to stress and promotes mental well-being.
  - *Anti-inflammatory*:
    - Contains compounds with anti-inflammatory effects.
  - *Antimicrobial Properties*:
    - Exhibits antimicrobial effects against certain pathogens.
  - *Blood Sugar Regulation*:
    - May help regulate blood sugar levels.

8. Milk Thistle (Silybum marianum):

- **Medicinal Properties**:
  - *Hepatoprotective*:
    - Protects and supports the liver, making it beneficial for liver conditions.
  - *Antioxidant*:
    - Exhibits antioxidant effects, supporting overall well-being.
  - *Anti-inflammatory*:
    - May have anti-inflammatory properties.

- *Cholesterol Regulation*:
    - Some evidence suggests a role in regulating cholesterol levels.

9. Peppermint (Mentha × piperita):

- **Medicinal Properties**:
    - *Digestive Support*:
        - Alleviates symptoms of indigestion, bloating, and gas.
    - *Headache Relief*:
        - Peppermint oil may help relieve tension headaches.
    - *Respiratory Health*:
        - Exhibits antimicrobial properties, benefiting respiratory health.
    - *Oral Health*:
        - Traditionally used for its antimicrobial effects in oral care.

10. Rhodiola Rosea:

- **Medicinal Properties**:
    - *Adaptogenic and anti-stress*.
- **Applications**:
    - Stress management and mental fatigue.
    - Support for mood and emotional well-being.
    - Potential benefits for physical endurance.

These highlighted medicinal properties and applications showcase the diverse health benefits offered by these powerful herbs. As with any herbal supplement, it's essential to consult with a healthcare professional to ensure its suitability for individual health needs and potential interactions with medications or existing health conditions.

3.2 Herbal Preparations

3.2.1 Different methods of preparing and consuming herbs (teas, tinctures, poultices, etc.).

There are various methods of preparing and consuming herbs, each tailored to extract and deliver the beneficial compounds in different ways. Here are some common methods:

1. Herbal Teas:

- *Preparation*:
    - Infusing dried or fresh herbs in hot water.
    - Commonly made with leaves, flowers, or seeds.
- *Consumption*:
    - Drink as a soothing beverage.
    - Varies in strength based on steeping time and herb concentration.
- *Examples*:
    - Chamomile tea for relaxation.
    - Peppermint tea for digestive support.

2. Tinctures:

- *Preparation*:
    - Extracting herbal compounds in alcohol or glycerin.
    - Requires several weeks of steeping.
- *Consumption*:
    - Taken in small dropper doses, often diluted in water or juice.
    - Fast absorption due to the liquid form.
- *Examples*:
    - Echinacea tincture for immune support.
    - Valerian tincture for relaxation.

3. Capsules and Tablets:

- *Preparation*:
    - Ground herbs are encapsulated or compressed into tablets.
    - Often involves the use of additional excipients.
- *Consumption*:
    - Swallowed with water.
    - Provides a convenient and controlled dosage.
- *Examples*:
    - Turmeric capsules for anti-inflammatory support.
    - Garlic tablets for cardiovascular health.

4. Infused Oils:

- *Preparation*:

- Soaking herbs in a carrier oil (e.g., olive oil) for an extended period.
    - Heat or sunlight may be used to enhance extraction.
  - *Consumption*:
    - Applied topically for massage or skin conditions.
    - Used in cooking for added flavor and health benefits.
  - *Examples*:
    - Calendula-infused oil for skin health.
    - Rosemary-infused oil for culinary purposes.

5. Poultices:

- *Preparation*:
    - Crushed or mashed herbs applied directly to the skin.
    - Often combined with a moistening agent like water or oil.
- *Consumption*:
    - Applied to the affected area.
    - Covered with a cloth or bandage to retain moisture.
- *Examples*:
    - Comfrey poultice for wound healing.
    - Mustard seed poultice for congestion relief.

6. Decoctions:

- *Preparation*:

- - Boiling tough plant parts like roots, bark, or seeds to extract compounds.
    - Requires a longer boiling time than herbal teas.
  - *Consumption*:
    - Consumed as a warm beverage.
    - Often used for more substantial plant material.
  - *Examples*:
    - Dandelion root decoction for liver support.
    - Cinnamon bark decoction for digestive health.

7. Salves and Balms:

- *Preparation*:
  - Infusing herbs in a carrier oil, then combining with beeswax to create a solid texture.
- *Consumption*:
  - Applied topically for skin conditions or as a protective layer.
  - Melted salves can be massaged into the skin.
- *Examples*:
  - Calendula salve for skin healing.
  - Arnica balm for muscle relief.

8. Herbal Syrups:

- *Preparation*:

- Extracting herbs in water and combining with sweeteners like honey or sugar.
    - Often includes a reduction process.
  - *Consumption*:
    - Taken by the spoonful.
    - Provides a palatable way to consume herbs.
  - *Examples*:
    - Elderberry syrup for immune support.
    - Thyme syrup for respiratory health.

9. Herbal Baths:

- *Preparation*:
  - Infusing herbs in hot water, which is then added to the bath.
  - Can include fresh or dried herbs.
- *Consumption*:
  - Soaking in the herbal-infused bathwater.
  - Absorption through the skin.
- *Examples*:
  - Lavender bath for relaxation.
  - Chamomile bath for soothing irritated skin.

These methods offer diverse ways to incorporate herbs into daily life, catering to individual preferences and health needs. The choice of preparation method often depends on the desired outcome, the properties of the herb, and personal preferences. Always consider individual sensitivities and consult with a healthcare professional, especially if using herbs for therapeutic purposes.

3.2.2 Practical tips for incorporating herbs into daily life.

Incorporating herbs into your daily life can be a delightful and healthy addition. Here are practical tips to make herbs a regular part of your routine:

1. Herbal Teas:
- *Tip*:
    - Keep a variety of herbal teas on hand.
    - Create a ritual around tea time for relaxation.
- *Examples*:
    - Sip chamomile tea before bedtime for better sleep.
    - Enjoy a cup of ginger tea after meals for digestion.

2. Cooking with Herbs:
- *Tip*:
    - Grow your own kitchen herb garden for easy access.
    - Experiment with different herbs in various cuisines.
- *Examples*:
    - Add fresh basil to salads, pasta, or pizza.
    - Infuse olive oil with rosemary for cooking.

3. Herbal Infused Water:

- *Tip*:
    - Enhance your water with herbs and fruits for flavor.
    - Use a large pitcher with a variety of herbs for a refreshing blend.
- *Examples*:
    - Mint and cucumber-infused water for a cooling effect.
    - Lemon and thyme-infused water for a zesty twist.

4. Herb-Infused Oils:

- *Tip*:
    - Create your own herbal oils for cooking or massage.
    - Use infused oils in salad dressings or drizzle over dishes.
- *Examples*:
    - Infuse olive oil with garlic for cooking.
    - Lavender-infused oil for a relaxing massage.

5. Herb-Infused Vinegars:

- *Tip*:
    - Make herbal vinegars for salad dressings or marinades.
    - Experiment with different herb combinations.
- *Examples*:

- Tarragon vinegar for a classic French vinaigrette.
    - Basil-infused vinegar for a flavorful marinade.

6. Herb-Infused Salts:

- *Tip*:
    - Mix herbs with sea salt for a custom seasoning.
    - Keep herb-infused salts in small jars for easy use.
- *Examples*:
    - Rosemary-infused salt for roasted vegetables.
    - Citrus and thyme-infused salt for fish dishes.

7. Herb-Infused Honey:

- *Tip:*
    - Infuse honey with herbs for natural sweetness.
    - Use in tea, on toast, or as a sweetener for desserts.
- *Examples*:
    - Lavender-infused honey for a calming treat.
    - Thyme-infused honey for a unique flavor.

8. Herb-Infused Butter:

- *Tip*:

- Mix chopped herbs into softened butter.
- Use as a flavorful spread or for cooking.
- *Examples*:
    - Parsley and chive-infused butter for potatoes.
    - Sage-infused butter for pasta or risotto.

9. Herb-Infused Syrups:

- *Tip:*
    - Make herbal syrups for beverages or desserts.
    - Experiment with sweet and savory combinations.
- *Examples*:
    - Mint syrup for refreshing cocktails or mocktails.
    - Lavender-infused syrup for drizzling on desserts.

10. Herb-Infused Ice Cubes:

- *Tip*:
- Freeze herbs in ice cubes for a burst of flavor.
- Use it in drinks or when cooking.
- *Examples*:
- Mint ice cubes for iced tea or lemonade.
- Basil ice cubes for adding to sauces or soups.

11. Aromatherapy with Herbs:

- *Tip*:

- Place dried herbs in sachets for a natural air freshener.
- Use essential oils derived from herbs in diffusers.
- *Examples*:
- Lavender sachets for a calming aroma in closets.
- Eucalyptus oil in a diffuser for respiratory support.

12. Herb-Infused Skincare:

- *Tip*:
- Make herbal facial steams or masks.
- Infuse oils with herbs for natural skincare.
- *Examples*:
- Chamomile facial steam for relaxation.
- Calendula-infused oil for soothing skin.

Incorporating herbs into your daily routine doesn't have to be complicated. Start with a few herbs that resonate with you and gradually expand as you become more familiar with their flavors and benefits. Whether it's in your culinary creations, beverages, or skincare routine, herbs can enhance your well-being in various ways.

Chapter 4: Holistic Approaches to Common Ailments

Holistic approaches to common ailments involve addressing health issues not just at the symptom level but by considering the interconnectedness of the mind, body, and spirit. These approaches often incorporate lifestyle modifications, natural remedies, and practices that aim to promote overall well-being. Here are holistic approaches to some common ailments:

1. Stress and Anxiety:
- **Holistic Techniques**: Practice mindfulness meditation, deep breathing exercises, and progressive muscle relaxation to manage stress.

- **Herbs**: Consider adaptogenic herbs like ashwagandha and rhodiola for their stress-relieving properties.
- **Lifestyle Changes**: Prioritize adequate sleep, regular exercise, and a balanced diet to support overall resilience.

2. Insomnia:

- **Sleep Hygiene**: Establish a consistent sleep routine, create a relaxing bedtime environment, and limit screen time before bed.
- **Herbs**: Explore herbs like valerian, chamomile, or lavender for their calming effects.
- **Mind-Body Practices**: Engage in practices like yoga nidra or guided imagery to promote relaxation.

3. Digestive Issues:

- **Dietary Changes**: Adopt a whole foods-based diet rich in fiber, fruits, and vegetables. Consider eliminating potential trigger foods.
- **Herbs**: Ginger, peppermint, and fennel can be used for digestive support.
- **Probiotics**: Incorporate probiotic-rich foods or supplements to support gut health.

4. Headaches and Migraines:

- **Hydration**: Ensure adequate water intake throughout the day.

- **Herbs**: Feverfew and butterbur are herbs that some people find helpful for migraine prevention.
- **Stress Management**: Identify and manage stress triggers through relaxation techniques.

5. Common Colds and Immune Support:

- **Nutrient-Rich Diet**: Consume a diet rich in vitamins and minerals, especially vitamin C and zinc.
- **Herbs**: Echinacea, elderberry, and garlic are traditional herbs believed to support the immune system.
- **Hydration**: Drink plenty of fluids to stay hydrated.

6. Muscle and Joint Pain:

- **Anti-Inflammatory Diet**: Emphasize foods with anti-inflammatory properties, such as fatty fish, turmeric, and ginger.
- **Herbs**: Arnica and comfrey salves are traditional remedies for topical use.
- **Physical Activity**: Engage in gentle exercises like swimming or yoga to promote flexibility and reduce stiffness.

7. Allergies:

- **Local Honey**: Some people find relief from seasonal allergies by consuming local honey.

- **Quercetin**: Consider foods rich in quercetin, a natural antihistamine found in apples, onions, and berries.
- **Neti Pot**: Use a neti pot with saline solution for nasal irrigation.

8. Skin Conditions (Eczema, Acne):

- **Dietary Changes**: Identify potential trigger foods and consider an anti-inflammatory diet.
- **Topical Remedies**: Calendula, chamomile, and aloe vera can be soothing for various skin conditions.
- **Stress Reduction**: Manage stress as it can exacerbate certain skin conditions.

9. Fatigue:

- **Balanced Diet**: Ensure you are getting a variety of nutrients through a well-balanced diet.
- **Hydration**: Dehydration can contribute to fatigue, so stay adequately hydrated.
- **Regular Exercise**: Engage in regular physical activity to boost energy levels.

10. Menstrual Cramps:

- **Herbal Teas**: Chamomile and ginger tea may have soothing effects.
- **Heat Therapy**: Use a hot water bottle or warm compress on the abdomen.
- **Mind-Body Practices**: Yoga and mindfulness may help alleviate menstrual discomfort.

General Considerations:

- **Consult Professionals**: Before starting any new regimen, especially if you have pre-existing health conditions or take medications, consult with healthcare professionals.
- **Individualized Approach**: Holistic approaches are often individualized, and what works for one person may not work for another. Listen to your body and adjust accordingly.

Holistic approaches to common ailments focus on empowering individuals to take an active role in their health through lifestyle choices, natural remedies, and mind-body practices. While these approaches can be beneficial, it's crucial to seek professional guidance when needed and to integrate holistic practices in a way that complements conventional medical care.

4.1 Stress and Anxiety

4.1.1 Herbs effective for stress relief.

Several herbs are known for their adaptogenic and calming properties, making them effective for stress relief. Here are some herbs that have traditionally been used for managing stress:

1. Ashwagandha (Withania somnifera):

- **Properties**:
    - Adaptogenic herb.
    - Supports the body's ability to adapt to stress.
    - May have anti-anxiety effects.

2. Rhodiola Rosea:

- **Properties**:
    - Adaptogenic herb.
    - Helps the body adapt to stress.
    - May enhance mental and physical performance.

3. Holy Basil (Ocimum sanctum):

- **Properties**:
    - Adaptogenic herb.
    - Traditionally used for stress management.
    - May have anxiolytic (anxiety-reducing) effects.

4. Chamomile (Matricaria chamomilla):

- **Properties**:
    - Mild sedative properties.
    - Calming and relaxing.
    - Often used for promoting better sleep.

5. Lavender (Lavandula spp.):

- **Properties**:
    - Calming and soothing aroma.
    - Traditionally used for relaxation and stress relief.
    - Often used in aromatherapy.

6. Passionflower (Passiflora incarnata):

- **Properties**:
    - Mild sedative properties.
    - Calming effects on the nervous system.
    - May help alleviate anxiety.

7. Valerian (Valeriana officinalis):

- **Properties**:
    - Mild sedative properties.
    - Relaxing effects on the nervous system.
    - Often used for improving sleep quality.

8. Lemon Balm (Melissa officinalis):

- **Properties**:
    - Calming and mild sedative properties.
    - Traditionally used for reducing stress and anxiety.
    - May help improve mood.

9. Rhubarb (Rheum palmatum):

- **Properties**:
    - Adaptogenic herb.
    - May help the body cope with stress.
    - Used traditionally in Traditional Chinese Medicine.

10. Ginseng (Panax ginseng):

- **Properties**:
    - Adaptogenic herb.
    - May enhance resilience to stress.
    - May help improve energy levels and focus.

11. Eleuthero (Eleutherococcus senticosus):

- **Properties**:
    - Adaptogenic herb.
    - Supports the body's response to stress.
    - May enhance endurance and mental performance.

12. Kava Kava (Piper methysticum):

- **Properties**:
    - Mild sedative and anxiolytic properties.
    - Traditionally used in Pacific Island cultures for relaxation.
    - Moderation is key due to potential liver concerns.

13. Catnip (Nepeta cataria):

- **Properties**:
    - Mild sedative properties.
    - Traditionally used for calming the nervous system.
    - Often used for promoting sleep.

14. Skullcap (Scutellaria lateriflora):

- **Properties**:
    - Mild sedative and nervine properties.

- Traditionally used for nervous system support.

- May help alleviate anxiety.

15. Oatstraw (Avena sativa):

- **Properties**:
  - Nervine tonic.
  - Traditionally used for nervous system support.
  - May help soothe and calm the body.

16. Tulsi (Ocimum tenuiflorum):

- **Properties**:
  - Adaptogenic herb.
  - Traditionally used for stress management.
  - May have calming effects.

17. St. John's Wort (Hypericum perforatum):

- **Properties**:
  - Mood-balancing properties.
  - Traditionally used for mild to moderate depression.
  - Interacts with certain medications; consult a healthcare professional.

It's essential to note that individual responses to herbs can vary. If you are considering using herbs for stress relief, it's advisable to consult with a healthcare professional, especially if you are pregnant, nursing, taking medications, or have pre-existing health conditions. Integrating stress-management practices such as mindfulness, exercise, and a balanced diet can also contribute to overall well-being.

4.1.2 Additional holistic practices for managing anxiety.

Managing anxiety involves a holistic approach that addresses the mind, body, and spirit. Here are some holistic practices that may help in managing anxiety:

1. Mindful Breathing and Meditation:
- Practice deep breathing exercises to calm the nervous system.
- Incorporate mindfulness meditation to stay present and reduce racing thoughts.
- Guided imagery or visualization can also be beneficial.

2. Yoga and Tai Chi:
- Engage in gentle physical activities like yoga or Tai Chi to promote relaxation.
- These practices combine movement, breath, and meditation to reduce stress.

3. Regular Exercise:
- Establish a regular exercise routine to release endorphins, the body's natural mood lifters.

- Exercise can be a powerful tool in managing anxiety.

4. Adequate Sleep:

- Prioritize quality sleep to support overall mental health.
- Maintain a consistent sleep schedule and create a relaxing bedtime routine.

5. Balanced Nutrition:

- Eat a well-balanced diet with nutrient-rich foods.
- Avoid excessive caffeine and sugar, as they can contribute to anxiety.

6. Herbal Remedies:

- Incorporate herbs with calming properties into your routine, such as chamomile, lavender, or passionflower.
- Consult with a healthcare professional before using herbal supplements.

7. Journaling:

- Keep a journal to express and process your thoughts and emotions.
- Write about your fears and worries to help gain perspective.

8. Limit Stimulants:

- Reduce or eliminate stimulants like caffeine and nicotine, which can exacerbate anxiety.

- Opt for herbal teas or decaffeinated alternatives.

9. Social Support:
- Connect with friends, family, or support groups.
- Share your feelings and experiences with others who may offer understanding and encouragement.

10. Mind-Body Practices:
- Explore practices like biofeedback or progressive muscle relaxation.
- These techniques can help you gain awareness and control over physiological responses to stress.

11. Aromatherapy:

- Use essential oils like lavender, chamomile, or bergamot for relaxation.
- Diffuse oils, add them to a bath, or use them in massage.

12. Limit News and Information:
- Limit exposure to news and information that may contribute to anxiety.
- Establish designated times to catch up on current events.

13. Acupuncture:
- Consider acupuncture, which may help balance the body's energy and alleviate stress.

- Consult with a qualified practitioner.

14. Art and Creativity:

- Engage in creative activities like painting, drawing, or crafting.
- Creative expression can be a therapeutic outlet for emotions.

15. Laugh and Practice Joy:

- Watch comedies, spend time with loved ones, or engage in activities that bring joy.
- Laughter and joy can have positive effects on mental well-being.

16. Holistic Therapies:

- Explore holistic therapies like massage, reiki, or acupuncture.
- These therapies focus on balancing energy and promoting overall well-being.

17. Mindfulness-Based Stress Reduction (MBSR):

- Participate in MBSR programs, which combine mindfulness meditation and yoga.
- MBSR has been shown to be effective in managing anxiety.

18. Self-Compassion Practices:

- Practice self-compassion and self-kindness.
- Challenge negative self-talk and cultivate a positive and understanding inner dialogue.

19. Nature Connection:

- Spend time in nature, whether it's a walk in the park or simply sitting in a garden.
- Nature has a calming effect on the mind.

20. Therapy and Counseling:

- Seek professional help through therapy or counseling.
- Cognitive-behavioral therapy (CBT) and other therapeutic modalities can provide valuable tools for managing anxiety.

Remember that managing anxiety is a personalized journey, and different practices work for different individuals. It's crucial to consult with healthcare professionals or holistic practitioners to create a comprehensive plan that suits your specific needs and circumstances.

4.2 Digestive Health

4.2.1 Herbs that support digestive function.

Several herbs are known for their ability to support digestive function. They can help alleviate common digestive issues, promote gut health, and enhance overall well-being. Here are some herbs traditionally used for digestive support:

1. Peppermint (Mentha × piperita):

- **Benefits**:
    - Relieves indigestion and bloating.
    - Calms muscle spasms in the gastrointestinal tract.
    - Supports the gallbladder and bile flow.

2. Ginger (Zingiber officinale):

- **Benefits**:
    - Eases nausea and vomiting.
    - Stimulates digestion and relieves indigestion.
    - Anti-inflammatory effects on the digestive tract.

3. Chamomile (Matricaria chamomilla):

- **Benefits**:
    - Soothes the digestive tract and reduces inflammation.
    - Relieves indigestion, bloating, and gas.
    - Calming and may aid in stress-related digestive issues.

4. Fennel (Foeniculum vulgare):

- **Benefits**:
    - Relieves indigestion and bloating.
    - Alleviates gas and supports overall digestive health.
    - Acts as a carminative to reduce abdominal discomfort.

5. Dandelion (Taraxacum officinale):

- Benefits:
    - Stimulates digestion and supports liver function.
    - Acts as a mild laxative and diuretic.
    - Rich in nutrients that support overall health.

6. Turmeric (Curcuma longa):

- **Benefits**:
    - Anti-inflammatory effects on the digestive system.
    - Supports liver function and bile production.
    - May help alleviate symptoms of irritable bowel syndrome (IBS).

7. Licorice (Glycyrrhiza glabra):

- **Benefits**:
    - Soothes the lining of the digestive tract.
    - Supports the adrenal glands.
    - May help alleviate symptoms of acid reflux.

8. Mint (Mentha spp.):

- **Benefits**:
    - Relieves indigestion and bloating.
    - Calms muscle spasms in the digestive tract.
    - Enhances bile flow for digestion.

9. Gentian (Gentiana lutea):

- **Benefits**:
    - Stimulates digestive juices and promotes appetite.
    - Traditionally used as a bitter tonic to support digestion.
    - May alleviate symptoms of indigestion.

10. Artichoke (Cynara scolymus):

- **Benefits**:
  - Supports liver function and bile production.
  - Aids in digestion and alleviates symptoms of indigestion.
  - Contains compounds that promote overall digestive health.

11. Marshmallow Root (Althaea officinalis):

- Benefits:
  - Soothes and coats the digestive tract.
  - Supports the mucous membranes of the stomach.
  - May help alleviate symptoms of heartburn.

12. Cardamom (Elettaria cardamomum):

- Benefits:
  - Aids digestion and reduces gas.
  - Has carminative properties to ease bloating.
  - Adds flavor to dishes and beverages.

13. Gentle Laxative Herbs (e.g., Senna, Cascara Sagrada):

- **Benefits**:
  - Provide mild laxative effects to relieve constipation.
  - Stimulate bowel movements gently.
  - Should be used with caution and under guidance.

14. Triphala:

- **Benefits**:
  - A traditional Ayurvedic blend of three fruits (Amalaki, Bibhitaki, and Haritaki).
  - Supports digestion, detoxification, and regular bowel movements.

15. Angelica Root (Angelica archangelica):

- **Benefits**:
  - Supports digestion and relieves indigestion.
  - Traditionally used as a digestive tonic.
  - May help alleviate symptoms of bloating.

16. Cumin (Cuminum cyminum):

- **Benefits**:
  - Aids digestion and reduces gas.
  - Enhances flavor in cooking.
  - Has carminative properties.

17. Coriander (Coriandrum sativum):

- **Benefits**:

- Aids digestion and reduces gas.
- Adds a citrusy flavor to dishes.
- Traditionally used in digestive tonics.

18. Aloe Vera:

- **Benefits**:
  - Supports digestive health.
  - May help soothe symptoms of irritable bowel syndrome (IBS).
  - Should be used in moderation.

19. Caraway (Carum carvi):

- **Benefits**:
  - Aids digestion and reduces bloating.
  - Adds a warm, slightly sweet flavor to dishes.
  - Traditionally used as a digestive aid.

20. Cinnamon (Cinnamomum verum):

- **Benefits**:
  - Supports digestion and helps alleviate gas.
  - Adds a sweet and warming flavor to dishes.
  - May help regulate blood sugar levels.

When incorporating herbs for digestive support, it's essential to consider individual sensitivities and consult with a healthcare professional, especially if you have pre-existing health conditions or are taking medications. Additionally, using a combination of herbs and maintaining a healthy lifestyle can contribute to optimal digestive well-being.

4.2.2 Dietary tips for maintaining a healthy gut.

Maintaining a healthy gut is essential for overall well-being. A balanced and diverse diet plays a crucial role in promoting gut health. Here are some dietary tips to support a healthy gut:

1. Eat a Diverse Range of Foods:

- Consume a variety of fruits, vegetables, whole grains, legumes, nuts, and seeds.
- Different foods provide different types of fiber and nutrients that contribute to a diverse gut microbiome.

2. Include Fiber-Rich Foods:

- Fiber supports the growth of beneficial gut bacteria.
- Include sources of soluble and insoluble fiber, such as whole grains, vegetables, fruits, and legumes.

3. Prebiotic-Rich Foods:

- Incorporate prebiotic-rich foods that feed beneficial bacteria.
- Examples include garlic, onions, leeks, asparagus, bananas, and Jerusalem artichokes.

4. Probiotic-Rich Foods:

- Include foods with natural probiotics to introduce beneficial bacteria.
- Examples include yogurt, kefir, sauerkraut, kimchi, miso, and kombucha.

5. Fermented Foods:

- Fermented foods support a healthy gut microbiome.
- Choose naturally fermented options without excessive added sugars or preservatives.

6. Limit Added Sugars:

- Excessive sugar intake may negatively impact gut health.
- Reduce consumption of sugary snacks, desserts, and sweetened beverages.

7. Moderate Alcohol Consumption:

- Excessive alcohol can disrupt the balance of gut bacteria.
- Consume alcohol in moderation, if at all.

8. Healthy Fats:

- Include sources of healthy fats, such as avocados, olive oil, nuts, and fatty fish.
- Omega-3 fatty acids support anti-inflammatory processes in the gut.

9. Hydration:

- Drink plenty of water to support digestion and maintain gut function.
- Herbal teas and infused water can add variety to your hydration routine.

10. Limit Processed Foods:

- Highly processed foods may contain additives that can impact gut health.
- Opt for whole, minimally processed foods whenever possible.

11. Mindful Eating:

- Practice mindful eating, paying attention to hunger and fullness cues.
- Chew food thoroughly to aid digestion and nutrient absorption.

12. Gluten Sensitivity:

- If sensitive to gluten, consider reducing or eliminating gluten-containing grains.
- Explore gluten-free alternatives like quinoa, rice, and gluten-free oats.

13. Lactose Intolerance:

- If lactose intolerant, choose lactose-free or alternative dairy products.
- Consider dairy alternatives like almond or coconut milk.

14. Limit Artificial Sweeteners:

- Some artificial sweeteners may affect gut bacteria.
- Use them sparingly, and opt for natural sweeteners like stevia if needed.

15. Regular Meals:

- Establish a regular eating schedule with balanced meals.
- Consistent meal times can help regulate gut function.

16. Whole Foods:

- Emphasize whole, nutrient-dense foods for optimal gut nourishment.
- Minimize reliance on highly processed and refined foods.

17. Herbs and Spices:

- Incorporate herbs and spices like ginger, turmeric, and garlic for their potential digestive benefits.

18. Bone Broth:

- Consider including bone broth, which may support gut health with its collagen and amino acids.

19. Low FODMAP Diet (if needed):

- For those with irritable bowel syndrome (IBS), a low FODMAP diet may be beneficial under the guidance of a healthcare professional.

20. Consult with a Healthcare Professional:

- If you have specific dietary concerns or digestive issues, seek guidance from a registered dietitian or healthcare professional.

Remember, individual responses to dietary changes can vary. It's essential to listen to your body and make adjustments that align with your unique needs and preferences. If you have specific health conditions or concerns, consult with a healthcare professional for personalized advice.

4.3 Immune System Boosters

4.3.1 Herbs known for their immune-boosting properties.

Several herbs are known for their immune-boosting properties, helping the body defend against infections and support overall immune function. Here are some notable herbs with immune-boosting potential:

1. Echinacea (Echinacea purpurea):
- **Benefits**:
    - Stimulates the immune system.
    - Traditionally used to prevent and shorten the duration of the common cold.

2. Astragalus (Astragalus membranaceus):
- **Benefits**:
    - Adaptogenic herb that supports immune function.
    - Used in Traditional Chinese Medicine to strengthen the body's resistance.

3. Garlic (Allium sativum):
- **Benefits**:
    - Antiviral and antibacterial properties.
    - Supports immune function and has cardiovascular benefits.

4. Ginger (Zingiber officinale):
- **Benefits**:
    - Anti-inflammatory properties.
    - Supports immune function and soothes the digestive system.

5. Turmeric (Curcuma longa):

- **Benefits**:
  - Anti-inflammatory and antioxidant properties.
  - Supports immune health and overall well-being.

6. Elderberry (Sambucus nigra):

- **Benefits**:
  - Rich in antioxidants.
  - Traditionally used for immune support and to reduce the severity and duration of colds and flu.

7. Licorice Root (Glycyrrhiza glabra):

- **Benefits**:
  - Antiviral and anti-inflammatory properties.
  - Supports immune function and soothes respiratory issues.

8. Oregano (Origanum vulgare):

- **Benefits**:
  - Antimicrobial and antioxidant properties.
  - Contains compounds like carvacrol that may support immune health.

9. Cat's Claw (Uncaria tomentosa):

- **Benefits**:
  - Immune-modulating properties.
  - Used traditionally for immune support in South American herbal medicine.

10. Andrographis (Andrographis paniculata):

- **Benefits**:

- Antiviral and immune-stimulating properties.

- Traditionally used for respiratory and immune support.

11. Ashwagandha (Withania somnifera):

- **Benefits**:

-Adaptogenic herb that supports overall health.

- May enhance immune function and reduce stress.

12. Mushrooms (Reishi, Shiitake, Maitake):

- **Benefits**

- Rich in beta-glucans, which may enhance immune function.

- Adaptogenic properties support overall health.

13. Holy Basil (Ocimum sanctum):

- **Benefits**:

- Adaptogenic herb with immune-modulating effects.

- Traditionally used for respiratory health.

14. Rosehip (Rosa canina):

- **Benefits**:

- Rich in vitamin C and antioxidants.

- Supports the immune system and overall health.

15. Cinnamon (Cinnamomum verum):

- **Benefits**:
- Anti-inflammatory and antioxidant properties.
- Supports immune health and adds flavor to dishes.

16. Nettle (Urtica dioica):

- **Benefits**:
- Rich in vitamins and minerals.
- Supports overall health and may have immune-boosting effects.

17. Thyme (Thymus vulgaris):

- **Benefits**:
- Antimicrobial properties.
- Supports respiratory health and immune function.

18. Sage (Salvia officinalis):

- **Benefits**:
- Antioxidant and anti-inflammatory properties.
- Traditionally used for immune support.

19. Dandelion (Taraxacum officinale):

- **Benefits**:

- Rich in vitamins and antioxidants.
- Supports overall health and immune function.

20. Green Tea (Camellia sinensis):

- **Benefits**:
- Rich in catechins with antioxidant properties.
- Supports immune function and overall health.

When incorporating herbs for immune support, it's essential to consider individual sensitivities and consult with a healthcare professional, especially if you have pre-existing health conditions or are taking medications. A balanced and varied diet, along with a healthy lifestyle, contributes to overall immune health.

4.3.2 Lifestyle factors that contribute to a strong immune system.

A strong immune system is crucial for overall health, helping the body defend against infections and diseases. Lifestyle factors play a significant role in supporting immune function. Here are key lifestyle practices that contribute to a strong immune system:

1. Balanced Diet:

- **Key Components**:
    - Eat a variety of fruits, vegetables, whole grains, lean proteins, and healthy fats.
    - Ensure adequate intake of vitamins and minerals, including vitamins C and D, zinc, and antioxidants.
    - Include probiotic-rich foods for gut health.

2. Regular Exercise:

- **Benefits**:
    - Regular physical activity enhances immune function.
    - Moderate exercise supports the circulation of immune cells and reduces inflammation.

3. Adequate Sleep:

- **Benefits**:
    - Prioritize quality sleep for immune system repair and regeneration.
    - Aim for 7-9 hours of sleep per night.

4. Stress Management:

- **Strategies**:

- Practice stress-reducing techniques such as meditation, deep breathing, yoga, or mindfulness.
- Chronic stress can weaken the immune system, so finding effective stress management strategies is crucial.

5. Hydration:

- **Benefits**:
  - Stay well-hydrated to support the body's overall functions.
  - Water helps transport nutrients and supports the elimination of toxins.

6. Maintain a Healthy Weight:

- **Benefits**:
  - Maintain a body weight within a healthy range.
  - Obesity can negatively impact immune function, so focus on a balanced diet and regular exercise.

7. Moderate Alcohol Consumption:

- **Guidelines**:
  - Limit alcohol intake to moderate levels.
  - Excessive alcohol can impair the immune system and disrupt sleep.

8. No Smoking:

- **Risks**:

- Avoid smoking and exposure to secondhand smoke.
- Smoking damages the respiratory system and weakens the immune response.

9. Good Hygiene Practices:

- **Habits**:
    - Practice good hygiene, including regular handwashing.
    - Proper hygiene reduces the risk of infections.

10. Social Connections:

- **Benefits**:
    -Maintain social connections and engage in positive relationships.
    -Social support contributes to overall well-being and can positively impact immune function.

11. Limit Exposure to Environmental Toxins:

- **Precautions**:
    - Minimize exposure to pollutants, chemicals, and environmental toxins.
    - Follow safety guidelines in your workplace and home.

12. Vaccinations:

- **Guidance**:
    - Stay up-to-date with recommended vaccinations.

- Vaccinations help prevent specific infections and contribute to overall immunity.

13. Sun Exposure for Vitamin D:

- **Considerations**:
  - Get moderate sun exposure for vitamin D synthesis.
  - Vitamin D plays a role in immune function, and deficiency may impact the immune response.

14. Moderate Caffeine Intake:

- **Recommendations**:
  - Limit caffeine intake, especially in the evening.
  - Excessive caffeine can interfere with sleep, affecting immune function.

15. Regular Health Check-ups:

- Routine:
  - Schedule regular health check-ups and screenings.
  - Early detection and management of health conditions contributes to overall immune health.

16. Practice Safe Behaviors:

- **Precautions**:
  - Practice safe behaviors to prevent injuries and accidents.
  - Accidents and injuries can stress the body and impact immune function.

17. Mindfulness and Relaxation Techniques:

- **Approaches**:
    - Incorporate mindfulness practices and relaxation techniques into daily life.
    - Mind-body practices can positively impact the immune system.

18. Limit Processed Foods:

- **Guidance**:
    - Minimize the consumption of highly processed and sugary foods.
    - A diet rich in whole, nutrient-dense foods supports overall health.

19. Maintain Oral Health:

- **Importance**:
    - Practice good oral hygiene to prevent infections.
    - Oral health is linked to overall immune function.

20. Compliance with Medications:

- **Adherence**:
    - Take prescribed medications as directed.
    - Managing chronic conditions effectively supports immune health.

Adopting a combination of these lifestyle factors contributes to a resilient immune system. It's important to personalize these practices based on individual needs, and consulting with healthcare professionals can provide guidance tailored to specific health conditions or concerns.

Chapter 5: Cultivating a Holistic Lifestyle

Cultivating a holistic lifestyle involves integrating practices, beliefs, and habits that address the well-being of the whole person—mind, body, and spirit. It's about recognizing the interconnectedness of various aspects of life and making conscious choices that contribute to overall health and balance. Here are key elements to consider when cultivating a holistic lifestyle:

1. Mindfulness and Presence:

- **Mindful Awareness**: Practice being present in the moment, whether through mindfulness meditation, mindful eating, or simply appreciating the current experience.

- **Gratitude Practices**: Cultivate a sense of gratitude by acknowledging and appreciating positive aspects of your life.

2. Nutrient-Rich Diet:

- **Whole Foods**: Prioritize a diet rich in whole, unprocessed foods, including a variety of fruits, vegetables, lean proteins, and whole grains.

- **Hydration**: Drink plenty of water throughout the day to support overall health.

3. Regular Physical Activity:

- **Exercise Routine**: Engage in regular physical activity that includes both cardiovascular exercises and strength training.

- **Mindful Movement**: Explore practices like yoga, tai chi, or qigong for mindful and gentle movement.

4. Adequate Rest and Sleep:

- **Consistent Sleep Schedule**: Establish a regular sleep routine with consistent bed and wake times.

- **Sleep Environment**: Create a comfortable and calming sleep environment to support restful sleep.

5. Stress Management:

- **Stress-Reducing Practices**: Incorporate stress-relief techniques such as meditation, deep breathing, or progressive muscle relaxation.

- **Time in Nature**: Spend time outdoors and connect with nature to promote relaxation and reduce stress.

6. Healthy Relationships:

- **Quality Connections**: Foster positive and supportive relationships with friends and family.

- **Communication**: Practice effective communication and active listening in relationships.

7. Spiritual Connection:

- **Spiritual Practices**: Engage in practices that nurture your spiritual well-being, whether through prayer, meditation, or connection with nature.

- **Values and Purpose**: Reflect on your values and purpose, aligning your actions with what brings meaning to your life.

8. Holistic Healthcare:

- **Preventive Care**: Prioritize preventive healthcare through regular check-ups, screenings, and maintaining a proactive approach to health.

- **Complementary Therapies**: Consider integrative and complementary therapies that align with your holistic values.

9. Creative Expression:

- **Creative Outlets**: Explore and engage in creative activities that bring joy and self-expression, such as art, music, or writing.

- **Mindful Hobbies**: Adopt hobbies that promote mindfulness and relaxation.

10. Mind-Body Practices:

- **Meditation**: Incorporate meditation into your daily routine for mental clarity and emotional balance.

- **Breathwork**: Practice conscious breathing exercises to reduce stress and promote relaxation.

11. Environmental Awareness:

- **Sustainable Choices**: Make environmentally conscious choices in daily life, considering the impact of your actions on the planet.

- **Natural Living**: Bring elements of nature into your living space, such as plants, to enhance well-being.

12. Continuous Learning:

- **Holistic Education**: Stay curious and continually educate yourself on holistic health practices, mindfulness, and other areas of interest.

- **Reflective Practices**: Engage in reflective practices, such as journaling, to deepen self-awareness.

13. Digital Detox:

- **Technology Boundaries**: Establish boundaries for technology use to prevent information overload and promote a balanced lifestyle.

- **Mindful Screen Time**: Use technology mindfully and consciously, with periods of intentional disconnection.

Cultivating a holistic lifestyle is a personal and ongoing journey. It involves self-awareness, intentionality, and a commitment to nurturing various aspects of your life. Remember that small, consistent changes can lead to significant shifts in overall well-being over time. Listen to your body, embrace balance, and find what practices resonate most with you on your holistic journey.

5.1 Mind-Body Connection

5.1.1 The importance of mental and emotional well-being

Mental and emotional well-being play a crucial role in overall health and are intricately connected to physical well-being. Here are key points emphasizing the importance of mental and emotional well-being:

1. Holistic Health:

- Mental and emotional well-being are integral components of holistic health.

- A balanced approach to health addresses not only physical aspects but also mental, emotional, and spiritual aspects.

2. Impact on Physical Health:

- Mental and emotional well-being significantly influence physical health.

- Chronic stress, anxiety, and depression can contribute to various physical health issues, including cardiovascular problems, weakened immune function, and digestive issues.

3. Resilience and Coping:

- Strong mental and emotional health enhance resilience in facing life's challenges.
- Effective coping mechanisms contribute to adaptability, reducing the negative impact of stressors.

4. Quality of Life:

- Mental and emotional well-being contribute to an individual's overall quality of life.
- Positive mental health is associated with greater life satisfaction, fulfillment, and a sense of purpose.

5. Relationships and Social Connection:

- Healthy mental and emotional states foster positive relationships.

- Social connections and emotional support are crucial for mental well-being.

6. Productivity and Performance:

- Mental and emotional well-being positively impact cognitive function, concentration, and productivity.

- A healthy mind contributes to better decision-making and problem-solving.

7. Prevention of Mental Health Conditions:

- Prioritizing mental and emotional health can contribute to the prevention of mental health conditions.

- Proactive self-care measures can reduce the risk
  of anxiety, depression, and other mental health
  disorders.

8. Emotional Intelligence:

- Cultivating emotional intelligence enhances self-awareness and interpersonal relationships.

- Emotional intelligence supports effective communication, conflict resolution, and empathy.

9. Mind-Body Connection:

- The mind-body connection underscores the influence of mental and emotional states on physical health.

- Practices like mindfulness and relaxation techniques contribute to overall well-being.

10. Life Satisfaction:

- Mental and emotional well-being contribute to a sense of life satisfaction and happiness.

- Positive mental health is associated with a more positive outlook on life.

11. Stress Reduction:

- Effective management of stress is crucial for mental and emotional health.

- Chronic stress can have detrimental effects on both mental and physical well-being.

12. Improved Sleep:

- Mental and emotional well-being positively impact sleep quality.

- Adequate sleep supports cognitive function, mood regulation, and overall health.

13. Self-Esteem and Self-Confidence:

- Positive mental health fosters healthy self-esteem and self-confidence.

- Confidence contributes to a proactive approach to life's challenges.

14. Empowerment and Personal Growth:

- A focus on mental and emotional well-being empowers individuals to pursue personal growth.

- Continuous learning, self-reflection, and resilience contribute to ongoing development.

15. Reduction of Stigma:

- Prioritizing mental and emotional health helps reduce the stigma associated with mental health conditions.

- Open conversations and awareness promote a more supportive and understanding society.

16. Emotional Resilience:

- Building emotional resilience helps individuals bounce back from setbacks.

- Resilience is a key factor in navigating life's challenges with a positive mindset.

17. Positive Habits and Lifestyle Choices:

- Positive mental and emotional well-being often aligns with healthy lifestyle choices.

- Regular exercise, balanced nutrition, and adequate sleep contribute to both mental and physical health.

18. Prevention of Burnout:

- Prioritizing mental and emotional health is crucial in preventing burnout.

- Recognizing and addressing signs of burnout early on is essential for sustained well-being.

19. Cultural and Societal Impact:

- A society that values and prioritizes mental and emotional health fosters a culture of compassion and understanding.

- Collective efforts to support mental health contribute to societal well-being.

20. Enhanced Emotional Well-Being:

- Emotional well-being encompasses self-awareness, emotional regulation, and the ability to navigate life's ups and downs.

- An emotionally healthy individual is better equipped to handle stressors and maintain a positive outlook.

In summary, mental and emotional well-being are foundational to leading a fulfilling and healthy life. Prioritizing these aspects contributes to resilience, positive relationships, and a sense of purpose, ultimately

enhancing overall well-being. Individuals are

encouraged to seek support, practice self-care, and

engage in activities that promote mental and emotional

health as part of their holistic approach to well-being.

5.1.2 Holistic practices for cultivating mindfulness.

Cultivating mindfulness involves developing a heightened awareness of the present moment, fostering a sense of clarity, calmness, and focus. Here are holistic practices to help you cultivate mindfulness:

1. Mindful Breathing:
- **Practice**:
  - Focus on your breath, paying attention to the sensation of each inhale and exhale.
  - Use deep, intentional breaths to anchor yourself in the present moment.

2. Meditation:
- **Practice**:
  - Set aside time for meditation, focusing on your breath, a mantra, or a guided meditation.

- Start with short sessions and gradually extend the duration as you become more comfortable.

3. Body Scan:

- **Practice**:
  - Direct your attention to different parts of your body, noticing any sensations without judgment.
  - Progressively move through each part, from head to toe or vice versa.

4. Mindful Walking:

- **Practice**:
  - Take a slow, deliberate walk, paying attention to each step and the sensations in your body.
  - Notice the environment around you without getting lost in thought.

5. Guided Imagery:

- **Practice**:
  - Close your eyes and imagine a peaceful scene or engage in a guided visualization.
  - Use all your senses to make the experience vivid and immersive.

6. Mindful Eating:

- **Practice**:
    - Eat slowly and savor each bite, paying attention to the taste, texture, and aroma of the food.
    - Be present and avoid distractions like screens.

7. Yoga:

- **Practice**:
    - Engage in mindful yoga, focusing on the connection between breath and movement.
    - Choose poses that encourage mindfulness and body awareness.

8. Journaling:

- **Practice**:
    - Keep a mindfulness journal to reflect on your thoughts and feelings.
    - Write down moments of gratitude and observations about your experiences.

9. Mindful Listening:

- **Practice**:
    - Practice deep listening without interrupting or formulating a response.
    - Pay attention to the speaker's words, tone, and non-verbal cues.

10. Nature Connection:

- **Practice**:
  - Spend time in nature, whether it's a walk in the park, sitting by a lake, or hiking.
  - Observe the sights, sounds, and sensations around you.

11. Mindful Technology Use:

- **Practice**:
  - Be intentional about your use of technology.
  - Take breaks from screens, and when using devices, do so with awareness rather than on autopilot.

12. Gratitude Practice:

- **Practice**:
  - Regularly express gratitude for positive aspects of your life.
  - Keep a gratitude journal or take a few moments each day to reflect on what you're thankful for.

13. Mindful Communication:

- **Practice**:
  - Be fully present during conversations.
  - Listen attentively, pause before responding, and choose words mindfully.

14. Loving-Kindness Meditation:

- **Practice**:
  - Cultivate feelings of love and compassion toward yourself and others.

- Repeat affirmations or phrases that promote kindness and well-being.

15. Breath Awareness in Daily Activities:

- **Practice**:
- Incorporate mindful breathing into daily activities like washing dishes or commuting.
- Use these moments as opportunities to center yourself.

16. Mindful Stretching:

- **Practice**:
- Engage in mindful stretching or gentle yoga stretches.
- Focus on the sensations in your muscles and the breath.

17. Silent Retreats:

- **Practice**:
- Consider attending a silent retreat to deepen your mindfulness practice.
- Disconnect from external stimuli for a period of self-reflection.

18. Mindful Art:

- **Practice**:
- Engage in artistic activities with full awareness.
- Whether drawing, painting, or crafting, focus on the process rather than the outcome.

19. Mindfulness Apps:

- **Tools**:
  - Use mindfulness apps that offer guided meditations, breathing exercises, and mindfulness reminders.
  - Apps can provide structure and support for your practice.

20. Mindfulness Workshops and Courses:

- **Learning**:
  - Attend mindfulness workshops or courses to deepen your understanding and practice.
  - Connect with a community of like-minded individuals.

Remember, mindfulness is a skill that develops over time with consistent practice. Experiment with different practices, find what resonates with you, and integrate mindfulness into your daily life at a pace that feels comfortable. Over time, you may find that mindfulness enhances your overall well-being and your ability to navigate life with greater clarity and presence.

5.2 Balanced Nutrition

5.2.1 Guidance on a holistic approach to nutrition.

A holistic approach to nutrition emphasizes nourishing the body, mind, and spirit through a balanced and mindful approach to food. Here are guiding principles for a holistic approach to nutrition:

1. Whole Foods Emphasis:
- Prioritize whole, minimally processed foods.
- Choose fruits, vegetables, whole grains, lean proteins, nuts, and seeds for a nutrient-dense diet.

2. Balanced Macronutrients:
- Include a balance of carbohydrates, proteins, and healthy fats in your meals.
- Adjust proportions based on individual needs, activity levels, and health goals.

3. Mindful Eating:
- Eat with awareness and presence.
- Pay attention to hunger and fullness cues, savor the flavors, and avoid distractions like screens during meals.

4. Hydration:
- Stay well-hydrated with water, herbal teas, and other hydrating beverages.

- Monitor individual hydration needs based on factors like climate, activity level, and health status.

5. Nutrient Variety:

- Aim for a diverse range of nutrients by consuming a variety of foods.
- Incorporate different colors, textures, and types of foods to ensure a broad spectrum of nutrients.

6. Individualized Nutrition:

- Recognize that nutritional needs vary among individuals.
- Consider factors such as age, gender, health status, and lifestyle when crafting a personalized nutrition plan.

7. Plant-Based Emphasis:

- Include a variety of plant-based foods, such as fruits, vegetables, legumes, and whole grains.
- Plant-based diets can provide a rich array of vitamins, minerals, and antioxidants.

8. Moderation and Balance:

- Practice moderation in all aspects of eating.
- Enjoy a balanced diet without extremes, recognizing that occasional treats can be part of a healthy lifestyle.

9. Seasonal and Local Foods:

- Incorporate seasonal and locally sourced foods when possible.
- Seasonal foods often offer optimal freshness and nutritional value.

10. Intuitive Eating:

- Listen to your body's hunger and fullness cues.
- Trust your body to guide your food choices and avoid restrictive dieting.

11. Digestive Health:

- Support digestive health with fiber-rich foods, fermented foods, and adequate water intake.
- Pay attention to how different foods affect your digestion.

12. Limit Added Sugars and Processed Foods:

- Minimize the intake of added sugars and highly processed foods.
- Choose whole, natural sources of sweetness when needed.

13. Mind-Body Connection:

- Recognize the connection between mental and emotional well-being and nutrition.
- Consider how stress, emotions, and mindset impact food choices and digestion.

14. Meal Planning and Preparation:

- Plan and prepare meals ahead of time, when possible.

- This promotes intentional food choices and reduces reliance on convenience or fast foods.

15. Herbs and Spices:

- Enhance flavor and nutritional value with herbs and spices.

- Many herbs and spices also offer potential health benefits.

16. Individual Food Sensitivities:

Be aware of individual sensitivities or intolerances.

- If needed, consider elimination diets or seek guidance from a healthcare professional.

17. Social and Cultural Considerations:

- Recognize the social and cultural aspects of food.

- Enjoying meals with others and celebrating cultural traditions can enhance the holistic experience of nutrition.

- **18. Connection with Nature:**

- Appreciate the connection between food and the natural world.

- Gardening, visiting farmers' markets, or participating in community-supported agriculture can deepen this connection.

19. Holistic Mindset:
- View nutrition as one aspect of overall well-being.

- Consider how food choices align with broader lifestyle and health goals.

20. Ongoing Education:

- Stay informed about nutrition and wellness trends.

- Continuously educate yourself about the nutritional value of different foods and the evolving science of nutrition.

Remember, the goal of a holistic approach to nutrition is to nourish the whole person—body, mind, and spirit. It involves fostering a positive relationship with food, promoting overall well-being, and recognizing that each individual's nutritional needs are unique.

5.2.2 Tips on incorporating herbs into a balanced diet.

Incorporating herbs into a balanced diet is a flavorful and healthy way to enhance the nutritional profile of your meals. Here are some tips on how to incorporate herbs into your daily diet:

1. Fresh Herbs in Salads:

- Add fresh herbs like basil, cilantro, mint, or parsley to salads for a burst of flavor.
- Experiment with herb-infused salad dressings using olive oil, lemon, and your favorite herbs.

2. Herb-Infused Oils and Vinegars:

- Create herb-infused oils or vinegars by steeping herbs like rosemary, thyme, or garlic in olive oil or vinegar.
- Use these infused oils for dressings, marinades, or as a finishing touch to dishes.

3. Herb Garnishes:

- Garnish your dishes with finely chopped fresh herbs just before serving.
- Sprinkle herbs on soups, stews, grilled meats, or roasted vegetables for added freshness.

4. Herb Butter or Compound Butter:

- Make herb-infused butter by blending softened butter with chopped herbs like chives, tarragon, or dill.
- Use herb butter to flavor steamed vegetables, grilled corn, or on top of cooked fish or chicken.

5. Herb Pesto:

- Create pesto using fresh herbs, garlic, nuts, Parmesan cheese, and olive oil.
- Use pesto as a pasta sauce, a spread for sandwiches, or a topping for grilled meats.

6. Herb-Infused Water or Tea:

- Make refreshing herb-infused water by adding mint, basil, or citrus herbs to your water.
- Brew herbal teas with varieties like chamomile, peppermint, or lemongrass for a soothing beverage.

7. Herb-Rubbed Meats:

- Make herb rubs with dried or fresh herbs, garlic, and spices.
- Rub the mixture onto meats before grilling, roasting, or baking for added flavor.

8. Herb in Smoothies:

- Add herbs like cilantro or parsley to green smoothies for a nutrient boost.
- Combine herbs with fruits and vegetables for a unique and vibrant flavor profile.

9. Herb-Infused Grains:

- Mix fresh or dried herbs into cooked grains like rice, quinoa, or couscous.
- This adds an extra layer of flavor to your side dishes.

10. Herb Dips and Sauces:

- Prepare herb-infused dips using Greek yogurt, sour cream, or hummus.

- Serve as a flavorful dip for veggies, crackers, or as a condiment for grilled meats.

11. Herb in Stir-Fries:
- Toss in fresh herbs like basil, cilantro, or Thai basil at the end of stir-frying for a burst of flavor.
- This works well with Asian-inspired dishes.

12. Herb-Crusted Fish or Chicken:
- Create a herb crust using breadcrumbs, grated Parmesan, and chopped herbs.
- Coat fish fillets or chicken breasts before baking for a savory and aromatic dish.

13. Herb-Infused Yogurt:
- Mix finely chopped herbs into plain yogurt for a savory twist.
- Use as a topping for baked potatoes, grilled vegetables, or as a dip.

14. Herb Soups:
- Incorporate fresh or dried herbs into soups and stews during the cooking process.
- Herbs like thyme, rosemary, and bay leaves add depth to broth-based dishes.

15. Herb in Breakfast:
- Add herbs to breakfast options like omelets, scrambled eggs, or avocado toast.
- Chives, dill, or basil can elevate the flavor of your morning meals.

16. Herb-Infused Rice or Pasta:

- Cook rice or pasta with a bundle of fresh herbs, like rosemary or thyme.
- The herbs infuse their flavors into the grains as they cook.

17. Herb Stuffed Vegetables:

- Stuff vegetables like bell peppers, tomatoes, or mushrooms with a mixture of fresh herbs, breadcrumbs, and cheese.
- Bake until the vegetables are tender and the filling is golden.

18. Herb Marinades:

- Create herb-based marinades for proteins like chicken, fish, or tofu.
- Let them marinate before grilling or baking for enhanced flavor.

19. Herb-Focused Snacks:

- Make herb-infused popcorn by tossing fresh herbs or dried herb seasoning into the mix.
- Roast chickpeas with herbs for a crunchy and flavorful snack.

20. Herb Infusions for Desserts:

- Infuse desserts with herbs, such as adding mint to chocolate-based treats or basil to fruit salads.

- The combination of sweet and herbal notes can be delightful.

Experimenting with different herbs and incorporating them into various dishes allows you to discover unique flavor combinations while reaping the potential health benefits of these aromatic plants. Don't be afraid to get creative and enjoy the diverse tastes that herbs can bring to your meals.

Conclusion

1. Empowering Readers

- **Summary of key takeaways.**

Here are the key takeaways from the discussion:

1. **Introduction to Holistic Healing Herbs**: Holistic healing herbs encompass a wide range of plants with potential health benefits for the body, mind, and spirit.

2. **Purpose of the Book**: "The Power of Holistic Healing Herbs: Ancient Remedies for Modern Ailments" aims to explore ancient herbal remedies for contemporary health issues, providing a holistic perspective on well-being.

3. **Relevance of Holistic Healing**: Holistic healing addresses the interconnectedness of the mind, body, and spirit, focusing on treating the root cause of health issues rather than just symptoms.

4. **Growing Interest in Holistic Approaches**: There's a growing interest in holistic health as people seek more natural, personalized, and comprehensive approaches to well-being.

5. **Limitations of Conventional Medicine**: Conventional medicine has limitations, and there's a

need for complementary activities, including holistic approaches, to address the complexity of health.

6. **Understanding Holistic Healing**: Holistic healing considers the whole person, integrating physical, mental, emotional, and spiritual aspects for optimal health.

7. **Holistic Approach to Health**: The holistic approach to health involves fostering balance, addressing root causes, and recognizing the interconnectedness of different aspects of well-being.

8. **Interconnection of Mind, Body, and Spirit**: The mind, body, and spirit are interconnected, influencing each other's well-being and requiring a holistic approach to achieve overall health.

9. **Historical Roots of Holistic Healing**: Holistic healing has historical roots in ancient civilizations, where herbs and natural remedies were integral to healing practices.

10. **Traditional Healing Systems**: Traditional healing systems like Ayurveda and Traditional Chinese Medicine emphasize the use of herbs for holistic health.

11. **Central Role of Herbs**: Herbs play a central role in traditional healing systems, offering a diverse array of medicinal properties and applications.

12. **Scientific Studies on Herbal Remedies**: Scientific studies support the efficacy of herbal remedies,

showcasing their potential benefits for various health conditions.

13. **Common Misconceptions about Holistic Medicine**: Common misconceptions about holistic medicine include viewing it as unscientific or solely reliant on alternative therapies.

14. **Powerful Herbs and Medicinal Properties**: Various powerful herbs, such as echinacea, astragalus, garlic, and turmeric, possess medicinal properties supporting immune health and overall well-being.

15. **Lifestyle Factors for a Strong Immune System**:Lifestyle factors, including a balanced diet, regular exercise, adequate sleep, and stress management, contribute to a strong immune system.

16. **Importance of Mental and Emotional Well-Being**: Mental and emotional well-being are integral to overall health, impacting physical health, relationships, and quality of life.

17. **Holistic Practices for Mindfulness**: Holistic practices for cultivating mindfulness include mindful breathing, meditation, body scans, and mindful eating.

18. **Holistic Approach to Nutrition**: A holistic approach to nutrition involves whole foods, balanced macronutrients, mindful eating, and considering individualized nutritional needs.

19. **Incorporating Herbs into a Balanced Diet**:
Incorporate herbs into your diet through fresh herbs in
salads, herb-infused oils, garnishes, herb butters, and
various culinary techniques.

20. **Key Takeaways for Balanced Living**: Embrace a
holistic lifestyle by integrating mindful practices,
nourishing your body with whole foods and herbs, and
recognizing the interconnectedness of your physical,
mental, and emotional well-being.

These takeaways offer a holistic perspective on well-
being, encouraging a balanced and mindful approach to
health that integrates ancient wisdom with modern
understanding.

- **Readers should explore holistic healing as a complementary approach to conventional medicine.**

Dear Readers,

As you embark on your journey toward well-being, we
encourage you to explore holistic healing as a
complementary approach to conventional medicine. The
integration of both perspectives can provide a
comprehensive and personalized path to optimal health.

Holistic healing embraces the interconnectedness of your mind, body, and spirit, recognizing that well-being is a multifaceted tapestry. By considering the whole person, holistic approaches address not only symptoms but also the root causes of health issues, fostering balance and harmony.

Here are a few reasons to consider exploring holistic healing alongside conventional medicine:

1. **Comprehensive Care**:

- Holistic healing complements conventional medicine by offering a more comprehensive approach to health. It considers the physical, mental, emotional, and spiritual aspects of well-being, promoting a more complete understanding of your unique health needs.

2. **Individualized Solutions**:

- Holistic practitioners take a personalized approach to your health, considering your unique circumstances, lifestyle, and preferences. This individualized attention can lead to tailored solutions that resonate with your specific needs.

3. **Emphasis on Prevention**:

- Holistic healing often places a strong emphasis on preventive measures. By addressing lifestyle factors, stressors, and imbalances before they manifest as illness, you empower yourself to proactively manage your health.

4. **Natural and Integrative Therapies**:

- Holistic healing incorporates natural and integrative therapies, including herbal remedies, mindfulness practices, and nutritional approaches. These can work in harmony with conventional treatments, offering additional tools for managing health conditions.

5. **Enhanced Quality of Life**:

- The holistic approach seeks not only to alleviate symptoms but also to enhance your overall quality of life. By addressing the root causes of health issues and promoting balance, you may experience improvements in various aspects of your well-being.

6. **Mind-Body Connection**:

- Holistic healing recognizes the profound connection between the mind and body. Practices such as meditation, mindfulness, and stress reduction not only support mental and emotional well-being but can positively impact physical health.

7. **Patient Empowerment**:

- Engaging in holistic healing empowers you to actively participate in your health journey. Through lifestyle adjustments, mindful practices, and self-care, you become a co-creator of your well-being.

8. **Open Communication with Healthcare Providers**:

- Open communication with both holistic and conventional healthcare providers fosters a collaborative and integrative approach. Sharing insights about your holistic practices allows for a more comprehensive understanding of your health.

Remember, holistic healing does not seek to replace conventional medicine but rather to complement it. The integration of these approaches can create a synergistic effect, providing you with a well-rounded toolkit for achieving and maintaining optimal health.

Explore, experiment, and find the balance that resonates with you. Your health journey is unique, and by embracing the holistic perspective alongside conventional medicine, you open the door to a more holistic, integrated, and empowered approach to well-being.

Wishing you a journey filled with vitality, balance, and holistic wellness.

Warm regards,

Dr. Robert E. Wright

2. The Journey Ahead

- **Invitation to readers to continue their exploration of holistic healing.**

Dear Readers,

The path to holistic healing is an ever-unfolding journey—one that invites you to explore the intricate connections between your mind, body, and spirit. As you embark on this transformative adventure, we extend an invitation to continue your exploration of holistic healing.

Consider this not only as an invitation but as a call to embrace the full spectrum of well-being. Here's why we encourage you to take the next steps:

1. Discover Your Holistic Potential:

- Delve deeper into the world of holistic healing to uncover the vast potential it holds for your overall well-being. Explore practices that resonate with you, whether it's herbal remedies, mindfulness, or integrative nutrition.

2. Nourish Your Mind, Body, and Spirit:

- Holistic healing offers a unique opportunity to nourish every facet of your being. Take the time to understand the interconnectedness of your mental, emotional, and physical health, and explore practices that contribute to a harmonious balance.

3. Expand Your Toolkit for Wellness:

- Your wellness toolkit is a dynamic collection of practices and approaches. By continuing your exploration of holistic healing, you add valuable tools—herbs, mindful practices, nutritional wisdom—that can enhance your resilience and vitality.

4. Embrace Holistic Living:

- Holistic living is an ongoing commitment to conscious choices that support your well-being. Dive into the principles of holistic nutrition, mindful movement, and stress reduction to create a lifestyle that nurtures and sustains you.

5. Connect with a Community:

- Joining a community of like-minded individuals can enrich your holistic journey. Share experiences, insights, and learnings with others who are on a similar path. A supportive community can be a source of inspiration and encouragement.

6. Explore Holistic Practices Across Cultures:

- Holistic healing is deeply rooted in diverse cultural practices. Explore ancient healing traditions from around the world, discovering the wisdom embedded in Ayurveda, Traditional Chinese Medicine, Indigenous knowledge, and more.

7. Integrate Mindfulness into Daily Life:

- Mindfulness is not just a practice; it's a way of being. Explore how you can integrate mindfulness into your daily life—whether it's in your meals, your interactions, or your moments of solitude.

8. Deepen Your Understanding:

- Knowledge is a powerful ally on your holistic journey. Deepen your understanding of holistic principles, herbal remedies, and mind-body connections. Read books, attend workshops, and stay curious about the vast terrain of holistic well-being.

9. Celebrate Your Progress:

- Every step you take on your holistic journey is a cause for celebration. Acknowledge the progress you make, both big and small. Celebrate the positive changes you experience in your health, mindset, and lifestyle.

10. Seek Professional Guidance:

- Consider consulting with holistic practitioners, herbalists, or integrative healthcare professionals. Their expertise can provide personalized guidance tailored to your unique needs and health goals.

Remember, your journey is unique, and there is no one-size-fits-all approach to holistic healing. It's about finding what resonates with you, what brings you joy, and what supports your well-being.

So, with an open heart and a spirit of exploration, we invite you to continue your journey into the realm of holistic healing. May it be a path filled with self-discovery, vitality, and a profound connection to the holistic tapestry of life.

With warm regards,

Dr. Robert E. Wright

Here are resources to further your learning on holistic healing, herbal remedies, and holistic well-being:

Books:

1. "The Herbal Medicine-Maker's Handbook" by James Green:

- A comprehensive guide to making herbal remedies, including tinctures, salves, and teas.

2. "The Holistic Herbal" by David Hoffmann:

- An exploration of herbal medicine from a holistic perspective, covering traditional and modern approaches.

3. "Mind Over Medicine" by Lissa Rankin, M.D.:

- Explores the mind-body connection and the role of thoughts and beliefs in health and healing.

4. "The Four Agreements" by Don Miguel Ruiz:

- A guide to personal freedom and spiritual growth, emphasizing ancient Toltec wisdom.

5. "The Complete Book of Ayurvedic Home Remedies" by Vasant Lad:

- Provides insights into Ayurvedic principles and practical home remedies.

Online Courses and Workshops:

1. HerbMentor (LearningHerbs.com):

- Offers online courses on herbalism, including medicine-making, plant identification, and holistic health.

2. Mindfulness-Based Stress Reduction (MBSR) Programs:

- Many institutions and instructors offer MBSR programs, integrating mindfulness into daily life.

3. Coursera and Udemy:

- Platforms offering courses on herbalism, holistic health, nutrition, mindfulness, and related topics.

Websites and Organizations:

1. American Herbalists Guild (AHG):

- A professional organization promoting the study and practice of herbalism.

2. National Center for Complementary and Integrative Health (NCCIH):

- A valuable resource for evidence-based information on complementary and alternative medicine.

3. World Health Organization (WHO) Traditional Medicine Resources:

- Provides global perspectives on traditional and complementary medicine.

4. The Chopra Center:

- Offers resources and courses on holistic well-being, mindfulness, and Ayurveda.

Podcasts:

1. The Herbal Highway:

- Explores herbalism, holistic health, and the cultural uses of plants.

2. The Wise Traditions Podcast by the Weston A. Price Foundation:

- Focuses on ancestral wisdom, holistic nutrition, and traditional healing practices.

3. The Mindful Kind:

- Explores mindfulness, stress reduction, and practical tips for integrating mindfulness into daily life.

Documentaries and Films:

1. "The Magic Pill":

- Explores the impact of a ketogenic diet on health and well-being.

2. "Heal":

- Investigates the mind-body connection and the potential for self-healing.

3. "The True Cost":

- Explores the impact of the fashion industry on the environment and well-being.

Herbalism and Plant Identification Apps:

1. PlantSnap:

  - Helps identify plants using visual recognition technology.

2. Herbalpedia:

  - A comprehensive herbal database with information on medicinal plants.

3. Flora Incognita:

  - An app for identifying plants in the wild.

Remember to critically evaluate information and consult with qualified healthcare professionals for personalized advice. These resources can serve as valuable guides on your journey toward holistic well-being and deeper understanding of herbal remedies.

3. Additional Tips

- **Practical Tips and Recipes:**

Here are some practical tips and recipes to help you

incorporate herbs into your daily life for holistic well-

being:

1. Herb-Infused Water:

- Make refreshing herb-infused water by adding mint, basil, or cucumber slices to your water. This adds a burst of flavor without added sugars.

2. Herb-Infused Cooking Oils:

- Create herb-infused cooking oils by steeping rosemary, thyme, or garlic in olive oil. Use these oils for sautéing or as a drizzle over roasted vegetables.

3. Fresh Herbs in Salads:

- Toss fresh herbs like cilantro, parsley, or dill into your salads for a burst of freshness and added nutritional benefits.

4. Herb Butter for Vegetables:

- Make herb butter by blending softened butter with chopped herbs like chives, tarragon, or rosemary. Use it as a flavorful topping for steamed vegetables.

5. Herb Tea Blends:

- Create your own herb tea blends by combining dried herbs like chamomile, peppermint, and lavender. Experiment with different combinations for relaxing or energizing teas.

6. Herb-Infused Vinegars:

- Infuse apple cider vinegar with herbs like thyme, oregano, or basil. Use the infused vinegar in salad dressings or as a marinade.

7. Herb Pesto:

- Make a versatile herb pesto by blending fresh basil, garlic, pine nuts, Parmesan cheese, and olive oil. Use it as a pasta sauce, sandwich spread, or dip.

8. Herb-Marinated Grilled Meats:

- Marinate meats with a mixture of chopped herbs, garlic, lemon juice, and olive oil before grilling for a flavorful and aromatic dish.

ii. Recipes:

1. Turmeric Ginger Tea:
- **Ingredients:**

- o 1 teaspoon grated fresh turmeric
- o 1 teaspoon grated fresh ginger
- o 1 teaspoon honey (optional)
- o Lemon slices (optional)
- **Instructions**:

  Steep turmeric and ginger in hot water for 5-7 minutes.

  Strain and add honey for sweetness.

- Garnish with lemon slices if desired.

2. Herb-Infused Quinoa Salad:

- **Ingredients**:
  - o Cooked quinoa
  - o Chopped fresh herbs (parsley, mint, cilantro)
  - o Cherry tomatoes, halved
  - o Cucumber, diced
  - o Feta cheese (optional)
  - o Olive oil and lemon dressing
- **Instructions**:
  - o Mix cooked quinoa with chopped herbs, tomatoes, cucumber, and feta.
  - o Drizzle with olive oil and lemon dressing.
  - o Toss well and serve.

3. Lavender Lemonade:

- **Ingredients**:
  - o 1 cup fresh lemon juice

- o 1/2 cup honey or agave syrup
  - o 2 teaspoons dried lavender buds
  - o 4 cups water
  - o Ice cubes
- **Instructions**:
  - o In a saucepan, combine honey, lavender, and 1 cup of water. Bring to a simmer and stir until honey dissolves.
  - o Strain the lavender-infused honey into a pitcher.
  - o Add fresh lemon juice and remaining water. Stir well.
  - o Chill in the refrigerator and serve over ice.

4. Rosemary Garlic Roasted Vegetables:

- **Ingredients**:
  - o Assorted vegetables (e.g., potatoes, carrots, Brussels sprouts)
  - o Olive oil
  - o Chopped fresh rosemary
  - o Minced garlic
  - o Salt and pepper to taste
- **Instructions**:
  - o Preheat the oven to 400°F (200°C).
  - o Toss vegetables with olive oil, rosemary, garlic, salt, and pepper.
  - o Spread on a baking sheet and roast until golden and tender.

Additional Tips:

- **Herb-Infused Honey:**

- Infuse honey with herbs like lavender, thyme, or rosemary by placing the herbs in a jar and covering with honey. Allow it to sit for a week, then strain the herbs. Use the infused honey in teas or as a sweetener.
- **DIY Herbal Seasoning Blend**:
    - Create a custom herbal seasoning blend by mixing dried herbs like basil, oregano, thyme, and garlic powder. Sprinkle on roasted vegetables, grilled meats, or pasta dishes.
- **Herb-Infused Coconut Oil for Skincare**:
    - Combine coconut oil with herbs like calendula, lavender, or chamomile for a soothing and aromatic herbal-infused oil. Use it as a moisturizer or massage oil.

Experiment with these tips and recipes to bring the benefits of herbs into your daily life. Whether through culinary delights or soothing beverages, herbs can add a touch of nature's goodness to your holistic well-being journey.

- **References and Further Reading**

Here are references and further reading materials to deepen your understanding of holistic healing, herbal remedies, and related topics:

Books:
- "Medical Medium Life-Changing Foods" by Anthony William:

    - Explores the healing properties of various fruits, vegetables, herbs, and spices.

- "The Complete Book of Essential Oils and Aromatherapy" by Valerie Ann Worwood:

    - A comprehensive guide to essential oils and aromatherapy for holistic well-being.

- "The Healing Power of Mindfulness" by Jon Kabat-Zinn:

- Discusses the role of mindfulness in health and healing.

- "The Web That Has No Weaver: Understanding Chinese Medicine" by Ted Kaptchuk:

  - Offers insights into Traditional Chinese Medicine and its holistic principles.

- "The Ayurveda Way: 108 Practices from the World's Oldest Healing System for Better Sleep, Less Stress, Optimal Digestion, and More" by Ananta Ripa Ajmera:

  - Introduces Ayurvedic practices for holistic well-being.

- "Herbal Antibiotics, 2nd Edition: Natural Alternatives for Treating Drug-Resistant Bacteria" by Stephen Harrod Buhner:

- Explores herbal remedies with antibiotic properties.

Websites:
- American Herbalists Guild (AHG):

  - https://www.americanherbalistsguild.com/

  - Professional organization providing information on herbalism and holistic health.

- National Center for Complementary and Integrative Health (NCCIH):

  - https://www.nccih.nih.gov/

  - Government resource offering evidence-based information on complementary and alternative medicine.

- HerbMentor (LearningHerbs.com):

- https://www.learningherbs.com/
- Online courses and resources on herbalism and plant medicine.

Research Journals:
- "Journal of Herbal Medicine"

  - A peer-reviewed journal publishing articles on the use of medicinal plants in traditional and modern medicine.

- "The Journal of Alternative and Complementary Medicine"

  - Focuses on integrative and complementary approaches to health and healing.

Documentary Films:
- "The Magic Pill" (2017):

- Explores the potential benefits of a
    ketogenic diet on health.

- "Heal" (2017):

  - Investigates the mind-body connection
    and the power of self-healing.

Online Courses:

- Coursera: "The Science of Well-Being"

  - https://www.coursera.org/learn/the-science-of-well-being

  - Yale University's course on the science of
    happiness and well-being.

- Udemy: "Herbalism :: Introduction & Medicine
  Making"

  - https://www.udemy.com/course/herbalism/

- A course on herbalism, covering introduction and medicine-making.

These resources provide a diverse range of perspectives on holistic healing, herbal remedies, and integrative approaches to health. Remember to explore and discern information based on your individual needs and interests.

THANK YOU FOR READING